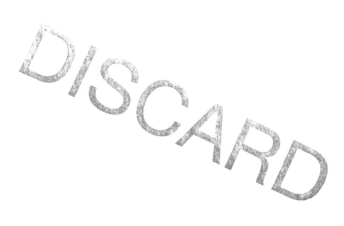

PARKINSON'S DISEASE

Nutan Sharma

Biographies of Disease
Julie K. Silver, M.D., Series Editor

GREENWOOD PRESS
Westport, Connecticut • London

Library of Congress Cataloging-in-Publication Data

Sharma, Nutan.
    Parkinson's disease / Nutan Sharma.
        p. ; cm.—(Biographies of disease, ISSN 1940-445X)
    Includes bibliographical references and index.
    ISBN-13: 978-0-313-34217-2 (alk. paper)
    1. Parkinson's disease. I. Title. II. Series.
    [DNLM: 1. Parkinson Disease. WL 359 S531p 2008]
    RC382.S477 2008
    616.8′33—dc22   2007048657

British Library Cataloguing in Publication Data is available.

Library of Congress Catalog Card Number: 2007048657
ISBN: 978-0-313-34217-2
ISSN: 1940-445X

First published in 2008

Greenwood Press, 88 Post Road West, Westport, CT 06881
An imprint of Greenwood Publishing Group, Inc.
www.greenwood.com

Printed in the United States of America

♾™

The paper used in this book complies with the
Permanent Paper Standard issued by the National
Information Standards Organization (Z39.48–1984).

10 9 8 7 6 5 4 3 2 1

To my son, Vikram E. Aldykiewicz, who is always patient and good-natured when his playtime gets interrupted by my work

Contents

Series Foreword

E very killer has a story to tell, and so it is with diseases as well: about how it started long ago and began to take the lives of its innocent victims, about the way it hurts us, and about how we are trying to stop it. In this *Biographies of Disease* series, the authors tell the stories of the diseases that we have come to know and fear.

The stories of these killers have all of the components that make for great literature. There is incredible drama played out in real-life scenes from the past, present, and future. You'll read about how men and women of science stumbled trying to save the lives of those they aimed to protect. Turn the pages and you'll also learn about the amazing success of those who fought the killer and won, saving thousands of lives in the process.

If you don't want to be a health professional or research scientist now, when you finish this book you may think differently. The men and women in this book are heroes who often risked their own lives to save ours. This is the biography of a killer, but it is also the story of real people who made incredible sacrifices to stop it in its tracks.

Julie K. Silver, M.D.
Assistant Professor, Harvard Medical School
Department of Physical Medicine and Rehabilitation

Preface

This book is intended to educate the reader about Parkinson's disease. The history of Parkinson's disease, what is known about the causes of Parkinson's disease, and medications used to treat it are discussed in detail. Current scientific and medical research and the state of promising new therapies, such as stem cells, are discussed using language that is understandable to the lay reader.

The book also contains numerous case studies that illustrate how those who have Parkinson's disease experience and cope with it. These case studies are drawn from actual cases that the author has encountered. However, names and other identifying characteristics have been changed to protect the privacy of those involved. The goal of these case studies is to put the reader in the shoes of someone with Parkinson's disease, to understand how it impacts daily life.

Introduction

Parkinson's disease is a chronic, progressive condition that affects one's ability to move. Until the early 1970s, there was no treatment for this disorder. In the last thirty-five years, there has been an explosion in the number of effective treatments for Parkinson's disease. As a result, people with Parkinson's disease now live more independent, active lives.

The goal of this book is to provide straightforward information to the general public about what is known about Parkinson's disease and its treatment. This book contains medical information, in plain English, describing what is known about the causes of Parkinson's disease, the way in which the disease affects one's daily life, and the current state of treatment. This book also discusses the current state of research in Parkinson's disease, including a discussion about the ways in which scientific and medical research is conducted. The impact of Parkinson's disease on the entire family is discussed. In addition, a list of resources from which more information can be obtained is provided.

Patient anecdotes are found throughout the book and are intended to illustrate the ways in which people with Parkinson's disease cope with the illness and continue to lead independent lives. As a neurologist specializing in movement disorders, I have had the privilege of developing long-term relationships with many patients and their families. It is a pleasure to share with them in the milestones of life: family weddings, the birth of grandchildren, and fiftieth year wedding anniversaries. It is a great privilege to work with patients and their entire families, to assist them in coping with illness, and to help them live as active and independent lives as possible.

Throughout this book, I have tried to illustrate what daily life is like for individuals with Parkinson's disease. I have also discussed the current state of research and the many exciting areas that are being pursued to have a better understanding of the causes of Parkinson's disease and to develop better treatments. It is my hope that readers of this book will become inspired to pursue careers in science and medicine, for there is much work yet to be done.

1

Parkinson's Disease Defined

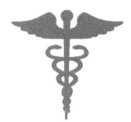

Parkinson's disease is one of many diseases that are collectively known as movement disorders. Movement disorders are neurological conditions in which a person slowly develops difficulty with the control of movements. Activities such as walking or holding a coffee cup may become difficult. In some cases, people cannot keep their body at rest, and some part(s) of the body remains in continuous motion.

Movement disorders can be divided into those that are hyperkinetic and those that are hypokinetic. Hyperkinetic movement disorders are those in which there is excess, uncontrolled movement. For example, some people have uncontrolled mouth movements, consisting of lip puckering or grimacing, when they are not speaking. Sometimes, these movements are so severe that they affect one's ability to eat. Uncontrolled mouth movements are one example of a hyperkinetic movement disorder and typically occur as a side effect of medication. The medications that are the most common cause of uncontrolled facial movements are the antipsychotics. Antipsychotic medications are used to treat people who have serious psychiatric disorders, such as schizophrenia. In a small percentage of people who take these drugs, excessive, uncontrollable movements of the face may develop.

Another hyperkinetic movement disorder that can be a side effect of taking antipsychotic medication is akathisia. Akathisia is a sensation of inner restlessness that makes a person feel compelled to move. A person with akathisia may get up and pace, after spending only a minute or so seated in a chair. Alternatively, a person with akathisia may stand in one place but constantly march the feet. Hyperkinetic movements that occur as a side effect of having taken psychiatric medications are referred to as "tardive" movements.

Chorea is another hyperkinetic movement disorder. Chorea is the brief contraction of muscles in the hands or feet that results in sudden, uncontrolled movements. A person with chorea may constantly move their fingers and hands, even when seated and reading a book, for example. Chorea and other hyperkinetic movement disorders can be seen as part of rare, genetic neurological disorders such as Huntington's disease and Wilson's disease.

Huntington's disease is a rare, inherited, progressive neurological disease in which affected individuals exhibit behavioral and personality changes, including chorea, dementia, and the inability to speak or swallow. These symptoms develop slowly, over years, and lead to death. There is no treatment for Huntington's disease.

Wilson's disease is a rare, genetic disorder in which copper accumulates in the liver and brain in affected individuals. Copper is found in most foods. Every cell in our body requires small amounts of copper to function properly. In most people, excess copper is secreted in the urine. In those who have Wilson's disease, copper begins to accumulate shortly after birth in first the liver and then the brain. Signs of the disease include liver damage, which is measured via blood tests, a variety of psychiatric problems including aggressive behavior, depression and suicide attempts, and hyperkinetic movements, including tremor and chorea. These symptoms usually begin to manifest in the adolescent years. Any teenager or young adult who has hyperkinetic movements should be tested for copper levels in both the blood and urine. Fortunately, treatment is available for Wilson's disease. It is easily treated with a medication that binds excess copper. Once the disease is controlled with treatment, people with Wilson's disease go on to live fairly healthy lives.

Hypokinetic movement disorders are those in which our ability to initiate movement, and move smoothly and easily, is affected. Rather than moving too much, people with hypokinetic disorders have trouble moving at all. Parkinson's disease is the most common type of hypokinetic movement disorder. In Parkinson's disease, the portion of the brain that helps to control the way we move loses some of its cells. The result is that the brain has a hard time sending messages to our body, telling our feet to start moving to walk and our arm to stop moving when we are sitting. Common symptoms of Parkinson's disease are that a person takes a longer period of time to stand up and start walking (called "hesitation") and when resting, an arm or leg shakes uncontrollably (called "resting tremor").

Parkinson's disease is a chronic, progressive disorder. Parkinson's disease typically progresses over a long period, in the range of ten to twenty years. It is not contagious. This means that one cannot develop Parkinson's disease by being close to someone else who has it. Infections do not play a role in the development of Parkinson's disease.

In only a few instances, Parkinson's disease is inherited from one's parents or grandparents. In the majority of cases, Parkinson's disease is not passed on from a parent to a child. If one's parent or grandparent has Parkinson's disease, there is no reason to be concerned that one is more likely to develop the disease. No one knows what the initial events are that cause a person to develop Parkinson's disease.

There are no laboratory tests that confirm the diagnosis of Parkinson's disease. A physician, typically a neurologist, examines someone over the course of two to three years to be certain of the diagnosis. This is because there are other movement disorders, similar to Parkinson's disease, that may have the same symptoms at first. It usually becomes clear over the course of two to three years whether someone has Parkinson's disease or a related disorder. The features that distinguish Parkinson's disease from related disorders will be discussed in Chapter 2.

In some people, Parkinson's disease develops slowly. In others, the symptoms develop more quickly. In some people, the symptoms are relatively minor. In others, the symptoms are more severe and disabling. The severity of the symptoms and the speed with which they worsen vary tremendously from one person to the next. There is a constellation of symptoms that people with Parkinson's disease may get. It is important to remember that not everyone is affected in the same way or to the same extent.

THE HISTORY OF PARKINSON'S DISEASE

Parkinson's disease is a condition that has been known about since ancient times. It is referred to in the ancient Indian medical system of Ayurveda under the name Kampavata. In Western medical literature, it was described by the physician Galen as "shaking palsy" in 175 AD.

The first modern description of Parkinson's disease, called *An Essay on the Shaking Palsy*, appeared in 1817 and was written by a London physician named James Parkinson. This established Parkinson's disease as a recognized medical condition. The essay was based on six cases he observed in his own practice and on walks around his neighborhood. He described what he observed in this way:

> The patient can [rarely] form any recollection of the precise period of its commencement. The first symptoms perceived are, a slight sense of weakness, with a proneness to trembling in some particular part; sometimes in the head, but most commonly in one of the hands and arms. . . . The propensity to lean forward becomes invincible. . . . As the debility increases and the influence of the will over the muscles fades away, the tremulous agitation becomes more vehement. (Parkinson 2002, 224)

The shaking or "tremor" is one of the four cardinal signs of Parkinson's disease (see Figure 1.1). The term "cardinal sign" refers to the physical features that are seen in the vast majority of men and women with Parkinson's disease.

The purpose of the essay was to encourage others to study Parkinson's disease in greater detail. About sixty years after James Parkinson's essay was first published, a French neurologist by the name of Jean Martin Charcot did exactly that. Charcot was the first physician to recognize the importance of Parkinson's work and named the disease after him. Since the late 1800s, a great deal has been learned about Parkinson's disease, yet much remains a mystery.

In the 1960s, scientists discovered that a dopamine deficiency in the brain is at the root of the disease, yet the events that lead to the dopamine deficiency are not at all understood even now. It was this discovery that led to the first effective medicinal treatment of the disease. In the 1960s, the drug levodopa was first administered to treat the symptoms and has since become the "gold standard" in medication.

Since the 1960s, research has continued to progress at a rapid rate. Despite the fact there is still no cure, the symptoms can now be effectively controlled and reduced in severity. The Parkinson's Disease Foundation was established in America in 1957 to assist sufferers and to fund and promote additional research. Several other foundations, dedicated to both the needs of people with Parkinson's disease and the financial support of research on Parkinson's disease, were established in the latter half of the twentieth century. A notable recent addition is the Michael J. Fox Foundation, named after the well-known television and movie actor. The goal of the Michael J. Fox Foundation is to develop a cure for Parkinson's disease within this decade.

Parkinson's disease affects people from every nation of the world. Parkinson's disease is one of the most common neurological diseases in North America. In the United States alone, more than 1.2 million people have

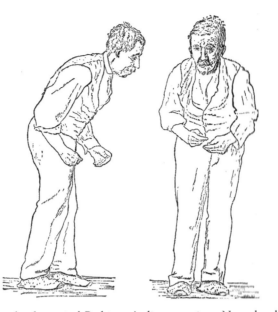

Figure 1.1. A sketch of a typical Parkinson's disease patient. Note the slightly stooped posture and tremor involving one arm. *From W. R. Gowers, A Manual of the Diseases of the Nervous System, Philadelphia, P. Blakiston, Son & Co., 1888.*

Parkinson's disease, and nearly 50,000 new cases are diagnosed each year. One of the many factors contributing to this phenomenon is that people are living longer. Our average lifespan has increased from fifty years in 1900 to an all-time high of seventy-seven years in 2001. Parkinson's disease is typically an illness of the middle and later years. Thus, it is not surprising that, as the proportion of Americans over the age of fifty-five grows, so will the number of Americans with Parkinson's disease.

THE ANATOMY OF PARKINSON'S DISEASE

The symptoms of Parkinson's disease develop because cells in the portion of the brain called the basal ganglia die.

Every portion of the brain plays a distinct and critical role. The brain cells that make up the basal ganglia are responsible for maintaining muscle tone and smooth, purposeful activity (see Figure 1.2). The basal ganglia control the activities that we normally perform without even thinking, such as walking. An abnormality in the basal ganglia results in poorly regulated movements and other signs that are discussed briefly below and in greater detail in Chapter 2 and throughout this book.

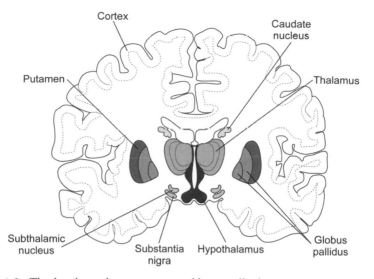

Figure 1.2. The basal ganglia are a group of brain cells that are interconnected with the cerebral cortex, thalamus, and brain stems. The basal ganglia are involved in motor control, emotions, and cognitive processes. The components of the basal ganglia are the caudate nucleus, the putamen, the globus pallidus, and the substantia nigra. *Illustrated by Jeff Dixon.*

Specific cells within the basal ganglia normally produce dopamine. Dopamine is one of many neurotransmitters produced in the brain. A neurotransmitter is a chemical that is released by one brain cell that then binds to a nearby brain cell. Once the neurotransmitter binds to the adjacent brain cell, it sets off a series of events within that cell. The second cell then communicates, by releasing a neurotransmitter, with a third brain cell. In this manner, cells in different parts of the brain communicate with each other and with the rest of the body.

Different cells, located in different parts of the brain, produce different neurotransmitters. Within the basal ganglia, there is a collection of cells called the substantia nigra. The cells of the substantia nigra produce dopamine, which plays an important role in sending signals to our body regarding movement. In Parkinson's disease, the cells of the substantia nigra die, resulting in the production of less dopamine than normal. As Parkinson's disease progresses, over many years, brain cells in the substantia nigra continue to die and levels of dopamine slowly decline.

POSSIBLE CAUSES

No one knows what sets off the death of the cells in the substantia nigra, although there are several hypotheses. One hypothesis focuses on the production of free radicals. Free radicals are substances that our body produces that can cause damage to cells if allowed to accumulate to high levels. Another hypothesis is centered on the potential role of environmental toxins in initiating the death of cells in the substantia nigra. Environmental toxins include any substance that gets into our body and causes damage. Environmental toxins may be in the air we breathe or the food that we eat, to name a few possible sources. Genetic factors, meaning the role that changes in the sequence of DNA that produces specific proteins may play, are also being studied as a potential cause or contributor to the initiation of cell death. Another hypothesis is that there is premature aging of the dopamine-producing brain cells, leading to their subsequent, early death and the development of Parkinson's disease.

Free radicals are molecules that are formed by every cell in the body as they go about their constant task of breaking down food, repairing injuries, and making the proteins needed to survive. Free radicals, if allowed to accumulate within a cell, have the potential to cause significant damage to the structures and proteins within that cell. One can think of each cell as a factory that produces energy and proteins that are needed to live. Free radicals are the unwanted, unhealthy byproduct of this factory, similar to the air pollution generated by a steel factory. Fortunately, every cell in our body can cope with and repair a small amount of damage caused by free radicals. Most of the free radical molecules are "mopped up" by being bound to other molecules, termed antioxidants. An antioxidant molecule binds to and stabilizes a free radical molecule, making it inactive. If an excess number of free radicals are produced or an inadequate number of antioxidant molecules are available, the free radical molecules will remain unbound and will damage other proteins within a cell. The process by which free radicals damage other molecules in a cell is called oxidation. If the oxidation process continues unchecked, in cells that are not able to stabilize the free radical molecules, an excessive number of proteins become damaged and accumulate inside the cells. If cells are filled with damaged proteins, they are unable to perform the functions vital to their survival and they die.

The free radical hypothesis of Parkinson's disease postulates that free radicals begin to accumulate, at very high levels, inside brain cells that make up the substantia nigra. The substantia nigra is one of the collections of brain cells that are part of the basal ganglia. This leads to excessive oxidation, with so much injury occurring within the cells of the substantia nigra that they cannot survive. If this hypothesis is true, then one way to limit the damage caused by oxidation may be to eat a diet rich in antioxidants or to take antioxidant vitamin supplements. Several antioxidant compounds have been or are in the process of being studied as potential treatments for Parkinson's disease. Treatment for Parkinson's disease will be discussed further in Chapter 4.

The hypothesis that environmental toxins are a cause of Parkinson's disease gained steam in the 1980s when several users of illicit drugs developed Parkinson's-like symptoms. These unfortunate individuals had injected themselves with a synthetic narcotic that had been produced illegally. The producers of the synthetic narcotic had inadvertently contaminated it with the compound known as MPTP (1-methyl-4-phenyl-1,2,3,6-tetrahydropyridine). MPTP has a chemical structure that is very similar to that of dopamine. As a result, MPTP is taken up and concentrated in dopamine-producing neurons within the brain. Within these brain cells, MPTP poisons the mitochondria. Mitochondria serve as batteries within each of our cells, producing the energy that cells need to survive. MPTP poisons the mitochondria, resulting in decreased energy production and cell death. The result is that dopamine neurons die, because these are the cells that allowed MPTP to cross their cell membrane. Cells in the rest of the brain, and most of the cells throughout the body, do not allow MPTP to enter and thus continue to function.

For the unfortunate individuals who injected themselves with a synthetic narcotic laced with MPTP, they developed signs of Parkinson's disease within a few days. Before this, they did not have any sort of movement disorder. This rapid onset of the symptoms of Parkinson's disease is unusual. The majority of people who develop Parkinson's disease are not users of illicit drugs. In most people, Parkinson's disease develops slowly, over several years, making it difficult to determine what caused the onset of the illness. In those illicit drug users who developed the symptoms of Parkinson's disease rapidly, shortly after injecting themselves with a synthetic narcotic, it was the combination of the speed with which they became sick and the fact that the illness occurred so quickly after taking the drug that led scientists to identify MPTP as toxic to dopamine-producing neurons. Since this discovery, MPTP has been used to generate models of Parkinson's disease in both rodents and primates. The importance of generating and studying animal models of Parkinson's disease, and any other human disease, is discussed in greater detail in Chapter 8.

Another hypothesis regarding the cause of cell death in Parkinson's disease focuses on genetic factors. Although there are only a few families in which Parkinson's disease is inherited, scientists hope that by studying these families we will learn principles regarding how dopamine cells die that can then be applied to all people with the disease. The contribution that our DNA makes to the likelihood of developing Parkinson's disease is being studied intensively. A more detailed discussion about the genetics of Parkinson's disease can be found in Chapter 3.

Scientists are also looking at the possibility that the dopamine-producing brain cells in people with Parkinson's disease age faster than normal. This theory is supported by the fact that the loss of antioxidant protective mechanisms is associated with both aging and Parkinson's disease. It is clear that the older one is, the more likely one is to develop Parkinson's disease. Thus, the factors that contribute to aging must also contribute to the likelihood of developing Parkinson's disease.

There are many factors that are known to contribute to aging. Based on extensive research done in yeast, it is known that the DNA in every cell is protected from degradation by telomeres. Telomeres are complex structures of DNA and protein that protect the DNA from damage. As a cell ages, the telomere becomes smaller. This results in less protection of, and therefore greater damage to, the DNA that encodes for proteins. Once the DNA is damaged, the proteins that are made based on the "recipe" provided by that sequence of DNA are not produced and/or do not function properly. A cell cannot function without proteins that work properly. Thus, excessive DNA damage leads to abnormal protein production and cell death. Massive cell death leads to failure of the organ in which the cells reside and subsequent death of the animal in which the organ is found. Because most of this work is occurring at a fundamental scientific level, in single-cell organisms such as yeast, it will not be reviewed in detail in this book. However, for those who are interested in this topic, several references regarding yeast and aging are listed in the bibliography (Laun et al. 2006; Kaeberlein, Burtner, and Kennedy 2007).

It is possible that scientists will discover that some or all of the mechanisms discussed here contribute to the development of Parkinson's disease. Scientists and physicians are aggressively exploring causes and possible treatments for Parkinson's disease. The National Institutes of Health (NIH), the government agency that supports biomedical research in the United States and in various countries throughout the world, supports a variety of research programs directed toward both understanding the cause of and finding new treatments for Parkinson's disease.

SIGNS AND SYMPTOMS

A "sign" of a disease is that which is evident to a physician during a physical examination. For example, a tremor at rest can be a sign of Parkinson's disease. A "symptom" of a disease is a subjective experience described by the patient. A symptom is not evident to an outside observer. For example, an aching muscle may be a symptom of Parkinson's disease (see Table 1.1).

Table 1.1.
The Signs and Symptoms of Parkinson's Disease

Signs	Symptoms
Bradykinesia	Aching muscles
Rigidity	Stiffness
Rest tremor	Hallucinations
Shuffling gait	Constipation
Dysarthria	Dysphagia
Drooling	
Masked facies	

There are four cardinal signs of Parkinson's disease: rest tremor, rigidity, bradykinesia, and balance difficulties. A tremor is a rhythmic, involuntary shaking of a part of the body. The rest tremor of Parkinson's disease typically begins in one hand or foot and is intermittent. The term "unilateral onset" is used to describe the usual pattern of onset in Parkinson's disease, in which the rest tremor begins on one side of the body and in one limb. You may have heard the tremor described as "pill rolling" because of the characteristic rolling movement of the thumb and opposing fingers. A person with a rest tremor does not exhibit a tremor with purposeful movement.

Jim is sixty-four years old and was diagnosed with Parkinson's disease six months ago. Jim does not like taking any type of medication. Although his neurologist gave him a prescription for medication to control his tremor, Jim has not started taking it. When Jim is seated in an armchair, he cannot control the continuous shaking of his right hand and forearm. When his wife, Amy, hands him a cup of coffee, he reaches out to grasp it in a single, smooth motion. Once his arm returns to rest on the chair, the tremor begins again and he spills some of the coffee. Jim and Amy have learned to compensate for this. Amy only fills the mug halfway with coffee and gives it to Jim in his left hand. Jim does not have a tremor in his left arm or either leg. Because Jim is doing well otherwise and has learned some "tricks" to minimize his chance of spilling coffee, he has decided that the bother of taking medication every day is not worth the potential benefit.

Gradually, over three to ten years, the rest tremor of Parkinson's disease will spread and may eventually affect all four limbs. Because the rest tremor disappears or decreases during movement, it does not interfere with the ability to perform tasks such as grasping objects. It is present in 70 to 80 percent of people with Parkinson's disease and may also appear in the face and jaw. A rest tremor is often more pronounced on one side of the body than the other and typically responds well to medication.

Clara is sixty-eight years old and was diagnosed with Parkinson's disease four years ago. When she was first diagnosed, she had a rest tremor in her left hand and arm. After seeing a neurologist, she began to take prescription medication three times a day. The medication controlled her tremor very well. No one else could see a tremor unless Clara became upset or anxious about something. About one year ago, Clara began to notice that her left leg and right arm would shake when she was seated or lying down. Also, the tremor in her left arm was only controlled for about three hours after taking each dose of medication rather than the full eight hours of control that she experienced before. Her neurologist prescribed a higher dose of medication and told her to take it four times a day rather than three times a day. The combination of taking both a higher dose of medication and taking it more frequently during the day resulted in good control of the tremor in both of her arms and her left leg.

Rigidity refers to stiffness that occurs in the arms or legs. It is not unusual for people with Parkinson's disease to first complain of soreness in an arm or leg, which they usually attribute to muscle strain. As the sensations of soreness and stiffness persist, it becomes clear that a more pervasive disorder is the underlying cause. Rigidity develops when the natural contraction and relaxation of opposing muscles fails to take place. Every muscle has a nearby muscle that opposes it. During normal movement, when one muscle contracts, its opposite muscle relaxes. Rigidity occurs when this balance is disturbed.

Bradykinesia means slowness of movement. In general, a person will complain of slowness in performing routine activities such as dressing, eating, and walking. Many people with Parkinson's disease never experience a rest tremor but do experience marked bradykinesia and rigidity. In addition to a loss of speed in Parkinson's disease, there is also a decline in the amplitude of repeated movements. For example, a person with Parkinson's disease takes smaller and smaller steps the farther he or she walks.

Miguel is seventy-two years old and lives with his son, Pablo, daughter-in-law, and three-year-old grandson. In the last two years or so, Pablo has noticed that his father has become slower in everything that he does. It takes longer for Miguel to shower and get dressed in the morning, it takes twice as long for him to finish a meal, and his daily walk in the neighborhood now lasts an hour rather than thirty minutes. At first, Pablo thought that his father was walking a longer distance. He then found out that Miguel was taking the same walk as he usually does, but it was taking twice as long to complete the same distance! At this point, Pablo realized that something was wrong and took his dad to the doctor.

The doctor listened to the history and found signs of rigidity and bradykinesia when he examined Miguel. The doctor suspected that Miguel had Parkinson's disease and discussed this possibility with both Miguel and Pablo. He then gave Miguel a prescription for medication to help alleviate these symptoms. Two months later, Miguel and Pablo returned for a follow-up visit. At this visit, Pablo told the doctor that he did notice a big change. Miguel could get ready more quickly in the morning. At meals, he only took five or ten minutes more than the others in eating. In general, other family members did not find that they were waiting for him as often as they had before he started to take the medication.

Clearly, Miguel benefited from taking the medication as prescribed by his doctor. The fact that he responded so well to the medication helps to confirm the diagnosis of Parkinson's disease.

Balance difficulties develop secondary to the fourth cardinal sign of Parkinson's disease, the loss of postural reflexes. Postural reflexes refer to our brain's ability to keep our body relatively straight and upright, whether we are on a boat, playing football, or sitting quietly in a chair. In particular, people with Parkinson's disease have a tendency to fall backward, usually because they do not lean far enough forward as they stand up. Thus, the center of gravity falls behind the feet, resulting in the tendency to lean backward and fall.

A number of secondary signs and symptoms can occur in people with Parkinson's disease. As stated above, not everyone with Parkinson's disease develops the same symptoms.

Masked facies refers to a loss of facial expression and a decreased rate of eye blinking. People with a masked facies appear to be staring intently at something. Their lips may be parted, and they do not smile or frown easily.

Dysarthric speech refers to the development of soft, slow, and slurred speech. Usually, the voice becomes soft, or low in pitch, early in the course of Parkinson's disease. As a result, someone with Parkinson's disease may have a harder time communicating on the telephone. As the disease progresses, speech tends to become slurred and even lower in volume. The worsening in speech can make it difficult to communicate with others even when seated together in the same room.

Parkinson's disease can affect the muscles involved in swallowing. A common problem early in the course of Parkinson's disease is dysphagia, which is difficulty in swallowing, with the food staying in the mouth for a longer period. In those who have had Parkinson's disease for a longer period, the muscles do not work in a coordinated fashion, and food may end up "going down the wrong pipe" into the trachea and lungs rather than into the esophagus and stomach.

Another symptom is drooling. Healthy individuals swallow unconsciously throughout the day, which allows the saliva in their mouths to enter the stomach. Because people with Parkinson's disease have difficulty in swallowing, saliva tends to build up in the mouth and can result in drooling.

There can also be gastrointestinal complications. Just as walking slows down in people with Parkinson's disease, the movement of the stomach and intestines slows down as well. The result is that food takes longer to travel through the body, resulting in a sensation of bloating and difficulty excreting stool.

In micrographia, handwriting becomes small because of difficulty with fine motor movement.

There can also be skin involvement. Increased sweating may occur and the skin may become oily.

Mental health issues can also be a sign. Depression is the most common psychological problem in Parkinson's disease. It affects about 40 percent of people with Parkinson's disease. Anxiety and cognitive disorders such as difficulty with multitasking may also occur. These are discussed in greater detail in Chapter 5.

2

The Diagnosis of Parkinson's Disease

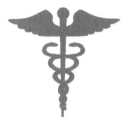

When the diagnosis of Parkinson's disease is suspected, it is important to find a neurologist who will assist in the confirmation of the diagnosis and prescribe treatment. A neurologist is a medical doctor who is trained to care for patients who have a disease of the nervous system. The nervous system comprises the brain, spinal cord, and nerves emanating from the spinal cord that control the muscles, organs, and other bodily structures. Some neurologists have additional training in the area of movement disorders, which is a subspecialty within neurology that focuses on diseases that affect one's ability to control movement.

Many large medical institutions house a center that specializes exclusively in movement disorders. Movement disorder centers provide specialized neurological care. They also usually provide specialized nursing care and evaluations by physical, occupational, and speech therapists. For people who live in rural areas, far from an academic movement disorders center, it can be helpful to travel there for an annual evaluation. The doctors, nurses, and therapists can devise a care plan that can be implemented by the doctors and therapists who are closer to where a given patient lives. In addition, for those patients who are interested in participating in research programs, most movement disorder centers are involved in multiple basic science, clinical research, and clinical medication trials at any given time.

NEUROLOGICAL EXAM

The most common initial signs of Parkinson's disease are rest tremor and/or bradykinesia. There may be less common symptoms as well, such as hypophonia, gait problems, and fatigue. Hypophonia is the term used to describe a weak voice that is low in pitch. It is typical for one of these symptoms to be present for months or even years before others develop.

At the doctor's office, the first step is to review the patient's medical history, medication history, and possible exposure to toxic compounds. It is important to review this information because some diseases, medications, and poisons can cause tremors that are similar, but distinct, from the rest tremor seen in Parkinson's disease. Hyperthyroidism, a medical condition in which the thyroid gland is overactive, is an example of an underlying illness that can cause tremor. Several drugs and toxins can also cause tremor: alcohol; caffeine; lithium (a drug used to treat bipolar disorder); antipsychotics (haloperidol [Haldol], chlorpromazine [Thorazine]); olanzapine (Zyprexa), which is a drug used to treat schizophrenia; metoclopramide (Reglan), a drug used to treat nausea; and valproate sodium (Depakene, Depacon), a drug used to treat epilepsy.

After reviewing the history, the doctor will proceed to the physical exam. Aspects of the exam that are unique to the evaluation of someone with a movement disorder include examining the muscles at rest and watching someone while they perform both fine motor tasks, such as tapping fingers together, and gross motor tasks, such as walking. To evaluate a rest tremor, a physician may use one of several techniques. The doctor may ask a patient to walk with hands relaxed alongside the body or to lie comfortably on an exam table. In both of these positions, the arms and hands are at rest and a tremor becomes more evident. To elicit a leg tremor, the doctor may ask a seated patient to cross his or her legs. This typically unmasks a rest tremor involving the leg that is on top.

Many symptoms of Parkinson's disease are unilateral. This means that one side of the body is more affected than the other. This is especially true early in the course of the disease, when a rest tremor or rigidity may only be found on one side of the body. The fact that the symptoms are unilateral may be obvious to the patient and family, but the doctor will want to confirm it by comparing both sides of the body during the exam.

To test for bradykinesia, the doctor may ask a person to open and close the fist, say ten times. Normally, in someone who does not have Parkinson's disease, the hand will open completely. The fingers spread and extend fully each time, and the hand opens to the same extent that it did the time before. In someone with Parkinson's disease, initially the fingers may be spread and open fully, but, with each subsequent try, the movement is less and less full. Instead of extending fully, the fingers bend. Rather than spreading apart, the fingers nearly touch each other. Another technique is to ask people to repeatedly tap their index finger and thumb together, making a circle. For someone with Parkinson's disease, repeated tapping results in a progressively slower movement, in which the finger and thumb have more difficulty meeting each other to tap and the size of the circle formed by the movement becomes smaller. Many patients with Parkinson's disease do not realize that their movements are incomplete. Frequently, it is friends or family members who notice these symptoms first. Decreased swinging of the arms during walking and a shuffling gait are related phenomena.

Slow movement is not unique to Parkinson's disease. Several other conditions can cause bradykinesia, and a doctor will want to rule them out. Other possible causes of slow movement include dementia, depression, arthritis, and "boxer's encephalopathy," caused by repeated head trauma

In dementia, people become slow because their ability to pay attention and focus on the task at hand worsens. For example, let's say that Jill is seventy-five years old and has moderate dementia. This means that she is able to live at home and bathe, cook, and clean for herself. However, she has stopped driving and does not go grocery shopping, because she cannot remember what she needs when she is walking in the aisles of the store.

Jill, her son, and daughter-in-law have been invited to a wedding to take place on Saturday evening. On Saturday afternoon, Jill needs to get ready. Her daughter-in-law calls at two o'clock to remind her that they will pick her up at five o'clock. Jill then takes her formal dress out of the closet and lays it on the bed before heading to the bathroom for a shower. She showers relatively quickly but then wanders around the house in her bathrobe, because she is not used to showering in the middle of the day and does not remember what she is supposed to do next. When Jill walks back into the bedroom, about twenty minutes later, she sees her formal dress on the bed and remembers that she must get ready for a wedding. She dries her hair, gets dressed, and gets her purse ready. By then, it is five o'clock. When the doorbell rings, Jill greets her son and daughter-in-law. Although she is fully dressed, her daughter-in-law notes that she is not wearing any makeup. Her daughter-in-law knows that Jill will be upset if she goes to the wedding without "her face on." Her daughter-in-law goes back to the bedroom with her, to help keep Jill focused and put her makeup on quickly.

In this case study, if a doctor were to ask Jill's son about her movements, he may well describe them as slow. This is because he knows that, when he was a boy, his mom used to get ready quickly and efficiently. It is shocking to him that now, even with three hours of preparation, his mom is not fully ready to leave the house. Based on this history, the doctor may become concerned that Jill is slow with walking and possibly has difficulty with fine motor movements, if she cannot put on makeup herself. However, by examining Jill and asking more questions of her family members, the doctor will be able to determine that Jill's slowness is attributable to difficulty in paying attention from dementia rather than from slowness of movement caused by Parkinson's disease.

Depression can also be confused with Parkinson's disease. Depression usually results in a lack of energy and lack of interest in participating in one's typical activities. Even getting out of bed in the morning and getting dressed can be hard to do. These relatively simple tasks may take much longer to complete when someone is depressed. In addition, depressed people may display a masked facies, because they no longer smile, laugh, or make eye contact when speaking to others.

Another disorder that can result in slow movement is arthritis. Arthritis is a term used to describe several medical conditions, in which there is degeneration of the joints. With age, the fluid that helps to lubricate our joints tends to dry up. This results in one bone grinding against another, which can be quite painful. Walking is affected when arthritis hits the knee or hip joints. Someone with arthritis in the hip and/or knees will walk slowly and carefully to minimize the pain felt with every step. However, their gait is usually wide based and the arms typically move normally. This is in contrast to the gait of Parkinson's disease, in which the steps are usually narrow based and the arms do not move very much. These features, among others, can help a doctor distinguish between the many different causes of slow movement.

Boxer's encephalopathy is the term used to describe brain damage that is the result of repeated head trauma. It is most commonly seen in professional boxers. The result is an individual who is "slow" in everything. He or she is slow to respond to questions, has trouble remembering facts, and is stiff and slow in all movements.

To accurately distinguish amongst the many potential causes of slow movements, it is essential to get the assistance of a doctor, particularly a neurologist. Typically, a neurologist can distinguish between Parkinson's disease, dementia, and boxer's encephalopathy relatively easily and quickly. However, there are several, relatively rare disorders that may resemble Parkinson's disease during the first few years in which someone has symptoms. These diseases are collectively known as the Parkinson's Plus disorders and are discussed in greater detail later in this chapter.

MAKING THE DIAGNOSIS

When a doctor sees a patient for the first time, it can be difficult to be certain that the proper diagnosis is Parkinson's disease and that the patient does not have one of several other disorders.

If a patient has a tremor, it is important to properly classify the tremor. A tremor is a rhythmic, involuntary shaking of a part of the body. The most common type is called an essential tremor. It occurs mostly in the hands, forearms, and head, when that part of the body is in motion or held in a specific position. The legs and torso are rarely involved. Essential tremor is often confused with the tremor of Parkinson's disease. The tremor of Parkinson's disease is called a rest tremor because it occurs when the affected body part is at rest and the muscles are relaxed. It is important to distinguish between different types of tremor for a doctor to prescribe the most effective treatment.

A thorough neurological exam can usually distinguish between a Parkinson rest tremor and the less serious essential tremor. Essential tremor is diagnosed in people who show a visible and persistent tremor that occurs when their arms or head are in a specific position or when they move. An essential tremor is not present when the arms are at rest. Although essential tremor tends to worsen with age, it is not associated with the other neurological symptoms that occur with Parkinson's disease, such as bradykinesia (slowness in movement) and loss of postural reflexes. Most cases of essential tremor are hereditary.

There is an array of disorders that resemble Parkinson's disease. These diseases are known collectively as the Parkinson's Plus syndromes and include multiple system atrophy (MSA), progressive supranuclear palsy (PSP), and diffuse Lewy body disease (DLBD). In the first one to two years after symptom onset, these disorders may mimic Parkinson's disease. This is why a neurologist typically follows patients over time to confirm the diagnosis of either Parkinson's disease or one of the Parkinson's Plus syndromes.

Those with MSA typically have a jerky, irregular tremor that does not resemble the pill-rolling tremor seen in Parkinson's disease. In addition, MSA is distinguished by the presence of urinary incontinence, reduced sweating, and a significant drop in blood pressure when a person stands up, which is referred to as orthostatic hypotension. In MSA, these symptoms occur within the first three to five years of disease onset. In someone with Parkinson's disease, in contrast, these symptoms may occur, but only ten to fifteen years after disease onset. Clinically, those with MSA do not experience an improvement in their symptoms when given dopamine replacement.

A characteristic of PSP is the inability to exercise voluntary movement of the eyes. For example, let's say that someone with PSP is watching a movie on a wide screen. The movie is a thriller and there is a scene in which the heroine is moving through a large, dark room. The audience member with PSP could not track the actor on the widescreen by simply moving their eyes across the screen. He or she would have to turn their head to keep the actor on the screen in their line of sight. Another feature of PSP is a marked change in personality; family members are quick to note apathy or inappropriate laughter in an affected individual. In some cases, family members first take their affected family member to a psychiatrist, thinking that the change in personality and behavior is attributable to mental, rather than neurological, illness. In addition, people with PSP have marked difficulty with gait and tend to have frequent falls within one or two years of developing symptoms. Thus, the gait difficulty in PSP develops much more quickly than the gait difficulty in Parkinson's disease.

Dudley Moore, a British comedian who was best known for his performance as a drunk millionaire in the 1981 film Arthur *was diagnosed with PSP at the age of sixty-four. The disease made it difficult for him to speak clearly and he was unable to walk safely. He was last seen in public two years later, at the age of sixty-six, when he received the Commander of the British Empire honor from Prince Charles. At that time, he was in a wheelchair and could not speak. Both his immobility and inability to communicate were caused by the progressive nature of PSP. A year later, he died from pneumonia that developed because of his limited mobility.*

There is also a form of dementia that has some of the motor features of Parkinson's disease. This type of dementia is known as DLBD. DLBD consists of a marked decline in intellectual function, visual hallucinations, and signs of bradykinesia, rigidity, and possibly rest tremor. In DLBD, the dementia and visual hallucinations progress rapidly within the first three years of symptom onset. The bradykinesia and rigidity progress more slowly. Unfortunately, treatment is limited because dopamine replacement, which would alleviate the motor symptoms of bradykinesia and rigidity, worsen the visual hallucinations and can produce an acute short-term worsening of the underlying dementia. DLBD is a disease entity that has been differentiated from other forms of dementia and formally studied only recently. As a result, information regarding the prevalence of DLBD is limited at this time.

One feature that is common to all the Parkinson's Plus syndromes is that the symptoms do not improve with dopamine replacement. This is in stark contrast to Parkinson's disease, in which the symptoms do improve significantly with dopamine replacement. It is this lack of response to dopamine, as well as the monitoring of the progression of symptoms, that helps to distinguish one of these syndromes from Parkinson's disease and from each other. Despite these identified variations in symptoms and the lack of response to dopamine, it can still be difficult to determine which of the Parkinson's Plus syndromes a particular individual has. The guiding principles outlined here are crude criteria for making a diagnosis within a group of poorly understood diseases.

Conventional laboratory investigations are not helpful in establishing the diagnosis of Parkinson's disease or any of the related disorders. Computed tomography and magnetic resonance imaging scans, which provide detailed anatomic information about the brain, do not reveal any consistent abnormalities in people with Parkinson's disease. An experimental imaging technique called positron emission tomography (PET) may be more helpful. PET examines blood flow and metabolism in the brain. Another experimental imaging technique is single photon emission computed tomography (SPECT). SPECT is used to examine blood flow in the brain and the activity of various receptors in the brain. At this time, both PET and SPECT are only done as part of specific research studies and are not available as standard clinical tests.

CLINICAL CHARACTERISTICS OF PARKINSON'S DISEASE

The most common signs of Parkinson's disease are rest tremor, bradykinesia, and balance difficulties. Rest tremor refers to rhythmic movement of a limb when it is in a relaxed, resting position. Bradykinesia refers to slowness in making movements. Balance difficulties refer to the tendency of Parkinson's patients to fall backward.

Gait and Balance Difficulty

The gait difficulty associated with Parkinson's disease typically consists of short, shuffling steps in which the heel is not placed completely on the floor. In addition, the head and shoulders are stooped, such that an individual has a tendency to look down rather than forward. Because of this posture, one's center of balance moves from its normal position, squarely between one's feet, to behind one's feet. This results in a tendency to lean and fall backward. In addition, the arms tend to stay stiffly at one's side rather than swing smoothly with the legs. Decreased arm swing also has a deleterious effect on one's ability to maintain a sense of balance while walking.

Dystonia

Dystonia refers to the uncontrolled contraction of counteracting muscles in any region of the body, such as a foot or arm. That means that the muscles that flex the arm will be active at the same time as the muscles that extend the arm. The result is a painful, twisted posture of the affected body part.

The most common form of dystonia in people with Parkinson's disease is seen as their medications wear off. At the end of a dose of medication, just before a person is due to take the next dose, one may experience foot cramping with an uncontrolled curling of the toes. This is a common problem that is caused by uncontrolled contraction of flexor and extensor muscles of the toes and sole of the foot.

Nonmotor Symptoms

In addition to difficulty with movement, people with Parkinson's disease have other symptoms, referred to as nonmotor symptoms. This encompasses all of the symptoms that are not related to movement. The nonmotor signs and symptoms of Parkinson's disease are numerous and not as well understood as the motor difficulties. These include cognitive dysfunction, sleep disturbance, urinary incontinence, sexual dysfunction, depression, and anxiety.

Cognitive Dysfunction

For the most part, people with Parkinson's disease retain their ability to process information and remember events and conversations. As the disease progresses, people may note that their thinking, just like their movements, may be slower during "off" periods. An off period is when the levels of dopamine in the brain are at a low point in the medication cycle. During an off period, one may take longer to respond to someone in a conversation or have a harder time concentrating while reading a newspaper article or book. Bradyphrenia is the term used to describe this slow thought process.

It is important to remember that bradyphrenia is distinct from dementia. Bradyphrenia occurs when one is "off." Dementia, conversely, is the persistent inability to form and retain new memories, retrieve old memories, and concentrate to perform complex tasks. Dementia is an abnormality in thinking that significantly impairs someone's ability to function on a daily basis. Bradyphrenia, conversely, is a short-term slowness in thought or worsening in the ability to respond to a question. Bradyphrenia improves when levels of dopamine are at a high point in the medication cycle, whereas dementia does not improve with dopamine treatment.

Another area in which cognition may be affected is in what is known as executive functioning. Executive function refers to our ability to set a goal and plan a method to achieve that goal, to switch from thinking and/or working on one task to working on another, and to think in the abstract.

Let's say, for example, that on a Monday you are invited to a barbecue and pool party on the coming Sunday. All of your friends will be there. The party starts at 3:00 P.M. and will include dinner. The problem is, you have to write a paper that is due on Monday, the day after the big party. Because your brain's ability to perform executive functions is intact, you quickly realize that the paper must be finished by Saturday, at the latest. To do this, you decide that you must make an outline by Wednesday, go to the library on Thursday, and then spend Friday afternoon and most of Saturday writing and revising the paper. By outlining and then following this plan, you are able to finish the paper by 3:00 P.M. on Sunday. You are then able to enjoy the party without a care in the world! However, perhaps you have a friend named Joe who has executive dysfunction. Joe handles this situation very differently. For example, Joe may decide that he simply cannot go to the party, or Joe wants to go to the party and starts to make an outline for the paper on Monday, the day he found out about the party. Then, on Tuesday, he gets a math assignment that is due on Thursday! Because people with executive dysfunction have trouble switching from one task to another, Joe spends Tuesday and Wednesday night working on the math assignment. On Thursday, Joe has an outline and not much else that is required to finish a paper before the party. Joe spends Friday afternoon and all of Saturday frantically researching and writing the paper. However, by Sunday morning, Joe is still in the midst of revisions. He is unable to complete the final version of the paper by 3:00 P.M. and so cannot attend the party after all.

In summary, people with executive dysfunction have trouble establishing and then meeting goals.

Urinary Incontinence

Urinary incontinence is the inability to control the flow of urine. The most common symptoms are increased urinary frequency and increased storage capacity of the bladder. Increasing frequency means that a person must urinate more often during the day. Increased bladder storage capacity occurs because the bladder cannot contract as well as it should. Thus, after every urination, the bladder still contains some urine. Because the bladder is never truly empty, it slowly expands over time. Urinary incontinence is a complication of Parkinson's disease and is seen in many other diseases as well.

People with Parkinson's disease have a tendency to urinate frequently. This can cause difficulty especially with sleep. Typically, the severity of urinary dysfunction tends to correlate with the severity of the underlying Parkinson's disease. The precise way in which the loss of dopamine-producing cells in the brain results in urinary problems is not understood.

Practical measures to help manage urinary incontinence include reducing evening fluid intake, emptying the bladder immediately before going to bed, and setting up a bedside commode. For those whose Parkinson's disease has progressed, making walking difficult, a bedside commode reduces the risk of falling because a person does not have to walk all the way to the bathroom, in the dark. For those who are also taking some heart medications, such as those that control blood pressure or stimulate urination, changing the time at which those are taken to earlier in the day may help reduce the need to urinate at night.

Sexual Dysfunction

In Parkinson's disease, according to the National Parkinson's Foundation, approximately 80 percent of men and 40 percent of women report experiencing diminished sexual activity. The problems with sexual function in Parkinson's disease can be caused by a variety of organic and psychological factors.

Some of the possible causes of sexual dysfunction in people with Parkinson's disease include psychological factors, medications, abnormalities of the autonomic nervous system, low dopamine levels in the brain, age and menopause, decreased ability to move, and dosing schedule for anti-parkinsonian medications.

Psychological factors that may affect sexual function include depression and anxiety. Depression, for example, is common in Parkinson's disease. Any symptoms of depression should be discussed with a physician. In addition, some medications that are used to treat depression have side effects related to reduced interest in sex, low sexual arousal, or the inability to attain an orgasm. This is especially true of some of the selective serotonin reuptake inhibitors (SSRIs, such as citalopram, fluoxetine, fluvoxamine, paroxetine, and sertraline). If depression is a factor, a psychiatrist can be helpful in finding the best antidepressant medication with the fewest sexual side effects. A more detailed discussion about depression and its impact on those with Parkinson's disease is found in Chapter 6.

Men with Parkinson's disease may experience erectile dysfunction, commonly referred to as impotence. Erectile dysfunction refers to difficulty in obtaining or maintaining an erection satisfactory for sexual intercourse. It affects approximately 30 million men in the United States and is estimated to be 1.6 times more common in men with Parkinson's disease than in men of the same age who do not have Parkinson's disease. The reason for erectile dysfunction in Parkinson's disease is uncertain, but there are a few possible explanations.

One theory regarding the cause of erectile dysfunction in Parkinson's disease is that it is caused by abnormalities in the function of the autonomic nervous system. The autonomic nervous system is the part of the nervous system that controls our organs in an involuntary, reflexive manner. For example, the autonomic nervous system controls our heart rate and blood pressure. When we start to run, our heart begins to beat faster and our blood vessels dilate, so that our muscles get more blood flowing to them. For the most part, the autonomic nervous system works without our conscious awareness.

An alternative theory is that erectile dysfunction in Parkinson's disease is directly related to the low dopamine levels in the brain. Experimental evidence suggests that dopamine may play a role in normal sexual functioning. Dopamine levels are abnormally low in people with Parkinson's disease, which may have an effect on sexual function as well as its more obvious effect on movement. Parkinson's disease is more common in older people, who may have other health conditions that limit their sexual activity. For example, diabetes, hypertension, and high cholesterol can cause erectile dysfunction.

Women with Parkinson's disease may experience decreased interest in sexual activity, a decreased level of sexual arousal, and reduced orgasm. A reduction in sexual arousal can interfere with normal vaginal expansion and lubrication, making intercourse uncomfortable. It is important to realize that these symptoms can have other causes, such as menopause or psychological issues. Most women who have Parkinson's disease have already reached menopause. Menopause refers to the normal end of menstrual cycles that occurs when a woman reaches her late forties. Thus, a fifty-five-year-old woman with Parkinson's disease may have reduced sexual arousal because of both menopause and her underlying disease.

Medical treatment for women is available. It includes but is not limited to treatment with the hormones estrogen, progestin, or testosterone. Because of the complexity of sexual function and dysfunction, it is best to seek a medical evaluation to determine the best treatment strategy.

Another complication for sexual activity is that Parkinson's disease can affect mobility, making it difficult to move around or roll over in bed. Reduced mobility may also be related to a person's dosing schedule for anti-Parkinson medications. Typical drug regimens are designed to produce optimal mobility in the morning and afternoon. The result is that people experience poorer motor function at night when they are more likely to feel like being intimate. A simple solution for some people would be to coordinate taking medications with sexual activity.

Concerning orgasm, a problem with reaching an orgasm is not as common in people with chronic disease as are problems with sexual desire or arousal. When difficulty does exist, it is usually related to a decrease in the intensity of the orgasm. Medications, particularly the SSRI antidepressants, can be the cause. High doses of alcohol can also interfere with orgasm.

Constipation

Constipation is a medical condition in which a person has hard stool that is difficult to excrete. Constipation is a frequent complication of Parkinson's disease. Just as the movements of one's limbs slow down, so does the motility of one's gastrointestinal tract. With the help of a physician, a personalized bowel regimen can be devised to ensure a daily, or every other day, bowel movement. Simple dietary habits, such as drinking six to eight glasses of water daily and eating fruit daily, can help to ensure a regular bowel movement. Medications, such as lactulose, that are not absorbed by the body and help to retain water in the colon can be prescribed. By retaining water in the colon, the stool that is formed will be softer and thus easier to excrete. The advantage in establishing a daily regimen to ensure regular bowel movements is that it minimizes the chances of becoming bloated and uncomfortable, which can interfere with one's level of energy and overall sense of well-being. It is important to remember that frequent use of laxatives is not recommended. Chronic laxative use can result in other health problems. A person with Parkinson's disease who finds that they need to use laxatives more than once per month should see their doctor to devise a better diet and medication regimen to prevent constipation.

Sleep Disturbances

Sleep disorders have been identified recently as a common problem in Parkinson's disease. It is not clear whether these sleep abnormalities are caused by the Parkinson's disease itself, a complication of the medications used to treat Parkinson's disease, or a combination of these two possible causes. Sleep disorders seen in those with Parkinson's disease include a sensation of restlessness while falling asleep, trouble staying asleep, vivid dreams, and daytime drowsiness. Research on sleep disorders in Parkinson's disease is in its infancy. However, a detailed discussion of the current state of knowledge in this area can be found in Chapter 5.

Sensory Abnormalities

People with Parkinson's disease may experience a variety of sensory symptoms, as well. A sensory symptom is one related to our five senses of touch, sight, hearing, smell, and taste. The sensation of touch includes the ability to sense light touch, such as a finger resting on one's leg, and pain.

At the onset of the disease, when the symptoms are mild and only one arm or leg might be affected, a person may experience a persistent, aching pain in that limb. This pain is usually caused by the persistent resting tremor in the affected limb. Fortunately, treatment with anti-Parkinson medications typically relieves this pain by controlling the tremor.

Another sensory abnormality that may occur early in Parkinson's disease affects the ability to smell. The loss of the ability to detect and discriminate odors is one of the most common symptoms seen in those with Parkinson's disease. The cause for this loss in the ability to smell is unknown. The medical term for the loss of smell is anosmia.

Within two to five years of being diagnosed with Parkinson's disease, some people may develop a variety of painful symptoms, such as tingling or burning in an arm or leg. Typically, the pain symptoms are most severe in the limb that is most severely affected by the Parkinson's disease. It is not clear whether increasing the anti-Parkinson medications relieve these symptoms of pain. To date, the underlying cause of these varied pain symptoms and the best way to treat them are not known.

Vision Problems

People with Parkinson's disease may also develop problems related to their eyes. These may include one or more of the following: dry eye, difficulty reading, or spasm of the eyelids. The most common problem in people with Parkinson's disease is dry eye with discomfort of the surface of the eye, resulting in a red, irritated eye. This is probably attributable to the fact that people with Parkinson's disease do not blink as often as healthy people. The result is that the surface of the eye becomes dry. Dry eye can be quite painful, and treatment is relatively easy with artificial tears or another similar medication recommended by an eye doctor.

Difficulty reading is challenging to evaluate because it can be caused by normal aging and the need for eyeglasses the Parkinson's disease, or both. Spasm of the eyelids, called blepharospasm (blepharo, eyelid; spasm, uncontrolled muscle contraction) can also be extremely frustrating. Blepharospasm is the uncontrolled contraction of the muscle within the eyelid, known as the pretarsal muscle, and the muscle that is just under the skin and surrounds the eye, known as the orbicularis oculi. It usually begins with excessive blinking and can be triggered by dry eye, bright light, fatigue, or stress. Sometimes people literally have to use their fingers to raise their eyelids. Spasm that becomes so persistent that it interferes with the ability to see can be treated with botulinum toxin injections.

Depression

Depression is common in Parkinson's disease. In fact, the National Parkinson's Foundation reports that about 40 percent of people with Parkinson's disease experience depression. You might say, "Well, it is probably depressing to have a chronic and debilitating disease." This is true. Many people with disabling disorders react by becoming depressed, but the truth is that depression is more common in Parkinson's disease than in other chronic illnesses. Interestingly, there is even evidence that depression can precede the onset of symptoms of Parkinson's disease. A detailed discussion of depression and other psychological aspects of Parkinson's disease can be found in Chapter 5.

The combination of signs and symptoms that can be found in cases of Parkinson's disease varies tremendously from person to person. It is important to remember that not every symptom discussed in this chapter will affect every person with Parkinson's disease. However, when someone with Parkinson's disease develops visual problems or unusual pain symptoms, it is important to keep in mind that these symptoms may be related to the underlying, chronic illness and not caused by a separate illness.

3

How Does Someone Get Parkinson's Disease?

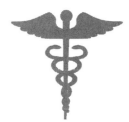

Before we begin a discussion of the possible causes of Parkinson's disease, there are two important facts to remember. First, no one is at fault when a person develops Parkinson's disease. Second, Parkinson's disease so rarely affects more than one person in a family that worrying about it occurring in multiple family members is pointless. However, the question of what are risk factors for Parkinson's disease is still a good one and one that researchers are trying to answer. A risk factor is defined as something that may increase the chance of developing a disease. For example, cigarette smoking is a risk factor for the development of lung cancer.

For many years, scientists have been trying to identify behaviors, toxins, genes, or anything else that might be risk factors for Parkinson's disease. As a result of the hard work of physicians and scientists over the last one hundred years, a few possible risk factors have emerged: genetics, environmental agents, and age. Studies looking at the distribution and causes of Parkinson's disease indicate that a combination of genetic and environmental factors may play a role in its development. The reason that age is called a risk factor is that the vast majority of people who develop Parkinson's disease are older; the average age of onset is sixty.

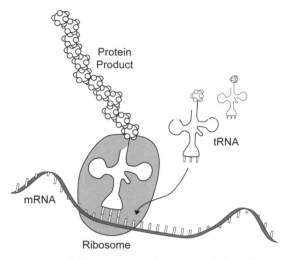

Figure 3.1. Proteins are made from a recipe that is encoded in the mRNA strand. The mRNA determines the order in which amino acids are put together. Next, tRNA molecules "read" the recipe of the mRNA and bring the right amino acid, at the right time, to the ribosome. The ribosome is the factory in which the amino acids are joined to make a protein. *Illustrated by Jeff Dixon.*

GENETICS AS A RISK FACTOR

Genetics is the study of heredity and how it varies from person to person. A gene is a specific portion of DNA, on a specific chromosome, that contains the instructions for the production of a specific protein.

Proteins are made up of individual units, known as amino acids. The DNA of each gene produces an mRNA strand. The mRNA is similar to a cooking recipe; it instructs the cell as to which amino acids should be put together, and in what order, to produce a specific protein (see Figure 3.1). Each human inherits a pair of genes for every protein produced in his or her body, with one gene coming from each parent. These genes become activated, in different cells and at different times during development, and direct the cell to produce a particular protein.

In the vast majority of cases, a specific protein produced in one person is the same as that protein produced in another person. This is because the protein is vital for our bodies to function properly.

In some instances, however, one or both of the genes that are inherited contain a mutation. A mutation refers to a change in the DNA sequence of a specific gene, resulting in a difference in the protein it produces. Sometimes, these mutations result in a protein that no longer functions. In other instances, a mutation results in a protein that functions in an abnormal way.

Mutations in several different genes have been identified in some families with Parkinson's disease. Each family, as discussed in detail below, has a mutation in a single gene resulting in the production of an abnormal protein. For some of these genes, every family member who inherits this mutated form of the gene develops Parkinson's disease. In the case of other gene mutations, only some family members who inherit the mutated form of a gene develop Parkinson's disease. Clearly, genetics plays a role in the development of Parkinson's disease in some people, but it is not the only factor that determines whether or not someone will develop Parkinson's disease.

Families with Gene-Related Parkinson's Disease

In a very few families around the world, an unusual number of members have Parkinson's disease. In these few families it is clear that Parkinson's disease has been passed down from one generation to the next. By studying these families, scientists have identified a number of different gene mutations that cause Parkinson's disease.

The first mutation that was identified was found in several generations of an Italian family, referred to as the Contursi kindred. The family originated in the town of Contursi, in the Salerno province of Italy. Sixty family members, over five generations, are known to have had Parkinson's disease. The cause of Parkinson's disease in the Contursi kindred is a mutation in the gene that produces a protein called alpha-synuclein. The gene mutation causes one change in the amino acid composition of the protein. Scientists do not know how the production of a mutated alpha-synuclein protein causes Parkinson's disease. This gene mutation is autosomal dominant, meaning that individuals need to inherit only one copy of the mutation to develop Parkinson's disease. This particular genetic defect is extremely rare and has been found in the Contursi kindred and in a few other families.

Mutations in alpha-synuclein are not the only way in which this protein results in Parkinson's disease. Another large family has been identified and studied, in which several members have developed early-onset Parkinson's disease. The term "early-onset" means that the symptoms of Parkinson's disease began before the age of forty. Scientists found that affected family members, meaning those who have Parkinson's disease, carry four copies of the normal gene for alpha-synuclein rather than the normal two copies. It appears that having an excess of the normal alpha-synuclein protein results in Parkinson's disease in this family. This discovery was made thanks to the work of numerous physicians and scientists over the course of the twentieth century. Neurologists first evaluated members of this family in 1920 and have continued to study healthy and affected descendants of this family for more than eighty years. In 2004, with the use of highly sophisticated techniques for identifying genes and genetic abnormalities, scientists at NIH discovered that the cause of Parkinson's disease in this family was the presence of an abnormally high number of copies of the normal gene for alpha-synuclein.

Early-onset Parkinson's disease has also been linked to the mutation of a second protein, named parkin. The normal parkin protein is thought to help identify other proteins within a cell that are damaged and need to be broken down. In a sense, the normal parkin protein acts as a marker to flag proteins that are damaged and must be cleared from inside the cell. In a survey of seventy-three families with early-onset Parkinson's disease, more than half produced an abnormal parkin protein. The current theory is that, when there is a mutation in parkin, damaged proteins fill the inside of a cell and cause the cell to die. However, many questions remain unanswered. For instance, why is it that a parkin mutation only results in damage to the dopamine-producing cells of the substantia nigra? Why isn't there cell loss in other parts of the brain and/or other organs of the body? Clearly, much more research needs to be done to understand what parkin, and a mutation in parkin, does in the human body.

A mutation in a third protein, called ubiquitin carboxy-terminal hydrolase L1 (UCH-L1), has been identified in a family in which multiple members have Parkinson's disease. UCH-L1, like parkin, is involved in the identification and breakdown of damaged proteins within brain cells. A mutation in UCH-L1 may lead to an accumulation of proteins within cells that results in their death. In the same way that some people have to clean their room before starting to study for a big test or work on an important essay, brain cells must stay "clean" to survive and function properly. If brain cells get filled with proteins that belong in the garbage, they cannot work and live.

This is a good example of how genetic research gives insight into how individual cells work. Although no one knows all the details of how a mutation in either the parkin or UCH-L1 protein causes Parkinson's disease, we do know that keeping brain cells free from damaged proteins is very important. This is a clue for the development of medication for the treatment of Parkinson's disease. Compounds that help to identify and break down damaged proteins may be helpful in treating people with Parkinson's disease.

Another clue that comes from the study of these mutations is that not everyone who has a mutation develops a particular disease. This is the phenomenon known as "penetrance." Penetrance is the extent to which the physical properties that are controlled by a specific gene will be expressed. If a gene has high penetrance, then the consequence of making the protein that this gene produces will always or almost always be apparent in the individual who has the gene. If a gene has low penetrance, then the consequence of making the protein that this gene produces will rarely be apparent in the individual who has that gene. For example, anyone who has a mutation in the alpha-synuclein gene develops Parkinson's disease. So, alpha-synuclein mutations have a penetrance of 100 percent. This is not true of all mutations. For instance, in families that have the UCH-L1 mutation, only some of the individuals with the mutation have Parkinson's disease. Other members of the same family, who have the same mutation, are disease free. Clearly there are other factors, which are currently unknown, that determine whether or not having the UCH-L1 mutation will result in the development of Parkinson's disease. Thus, the UCH-L1 mutation is referred to as having "reduced penetrance."

The mutations described above probably cause Parkinson's disease in only a few families. However, one genetic mutation has been identified, termed LRKK2, which is responsible for 5 to 20 percent of all the cases of Parkinson's disease that do run in families throughout the world. Multiple mutations have been identified in the gene LRRK2, which encodes the protein called leucine-rich repeat kinase 2. Although the way in which mutations in the LRRK2 gene result in Parkinson's disease is not known, it is interesting to note that more than one mutation in this gene exists and results in Parkinson's disease. Clearly, the protein produced by the LRRK2 gene is important in brain cells that produce dopamine. Without a proper LRRK2 gene, dopamine-producing brain cells do not survive, and the individual with the LRRK2 gene mutation develops Parkinson's disease.

Scientists hope that, by studying how Parkinson's disease develops in those rare families with genetic mutations, they will obtain information that helps everyone with Parkinson's disease. How could this happen? For instance, information already gathered concerning the function of the parkin and UCH-L1 genes has led some scientists, physicians, and pharmaceutical companies to study drugs that help keep brain cells clear of damaged proteins. Still other scientists are working on methods to turn off, or silence, certain genes. This may be useful in treating those people who have extra copies of the alpha-synuclein gene or other genes that may be identified as causing Parkinson's disease if more than two copies of the gene are present.

This fairly extensive discussion of the genetics of Parkinson's disease may make the reader worried about his or her own risk of developing Parkinson's disease. It is important to remember that the majority of these mutations have been identified in only a handful of families, in which several members have Parkinson's disease. In the vast majority of cases, Parkinson's disease develops in an individual who has no family history of the disease. So, if your parent or grandparent has Parkinson's disease, there is no need to worry about your risk of developing Parkinson's disease.

ENVIRONMENTAL RISK FACTORS

There have been suggestions that substances in our environment might increase the risk of developing Parkinson's disease. A number of industrial byproducts have been implicated as contributing to the risk of developing Parkinson's disease. These byproducts include copper, lead, manganese, mercury, and zinc. I use the term "implicated" because a clear relationship between exposure to a specific metal and the development of Parkinson's disease has been studied infrequently and only in small populations. These limitations make it difficult to establish a definite cause-and-effect relationship between exposure to a specific metal and the development of Parkinson's disease.

However, one unfortunate event does demonstrate that "Parkinson's-like" symptoms can be the result of exposure to a specific toxin. In 1982, in the San Francisco Bay Area of California, heroin users injected themselves with a synthetic narcotic that was contaminated by a chemical known as MPTP. The compound killed dopamine-producing brain cells and caused instant, severe, and permanent symptoms that looked like Parkinson's disease. The clinical effects of injecting MPTP were discussed in greater detail in Chapter 1. From the perspective of a scientist, this experience lends credence to the theory that exposure to certain toxic agents may cause Parkinson's disease. In addition, MPTP has been used to generate and study animal models of Parkinson's disease. The utility of animal models in the study of Parkinson's disease, as well as other human diseases, is discussed in greater detail in Chapter 8.

Other environmental risk factors that have been implicated in the development of Parkinson's disease are pesticides and herbicides. Pesticides are substances that destroy any living organism, whether it is a plant or animal, that is considered to be a pest. A pest is any living organism that is considered to be undesirable. Herbicides are substances that are specifically meant to kill unwanted plant growth. Several studies have associated pesticide and herbicide use with an increased risk of Parkinson's disease. However, the relationship between exposure to these chemicals and the development of Parkinson's disease is poorly understood. Specifically, studies of the effects of pesticides and herbicides involve the short-term exposure of rodents to relatively high levels of the chemical in question. It is difficult to then translate the results of this work to real-world exposure, in which humans are exposed to relatively low levels of these chemicals over many years.

Researchers have focused on the effect of herbicides and pesticides that have a chemical structure similar to that of MPTP. This focus is because MPTP has been identified as a toxin that results in the death of dopamine-producing neurons, as discussed in Chapter 1. One such herbicide is called paraquat. Paraquat is one of the most widely used herbicides in the world. Adult mice that were exposed to paraquat as newborns had decreased brain dopamine levels. However, these mice did not display overt signs of Parkinson's disease. In addition, most newborn human babies are protected from exposure to herbicides and pesticides. Thus, it is not clear how to translate the results of paraquat exposure in newborn mice into the potential risk of developing Parkinson's disease in adult humans, who are exposed to relatively low levels of paraquat for longer periods. To date, no herbicide or pesticide has been identified as clearly causing Parkinson's disease. Thus, there is no evidence to suggest that the routine use of herbicides on one's lawn or garden, using the precautions recommended by the manufacturer to minimize exposure, increases the risk of developing Parkinson's disease.

AGING AS A TRUE RISK FACTOR

The only known risk factor for developing Parkinson's disease is aging. The prevalence of Parkinson's disease, meaning the total number of cases of Parkinson's disease in a specific population at a given time, increases up to the ninth decade (ages eighty to eighty-nine) of life. At this time, information regarding the prevalence of Parkinson's disease beyond the ninth decade is not available. The relationship between Parkinson's disease and old age correlates with the normal changes in brain chemistry that occur with growing older, too. The number of cell receptors for dopamine, the neurotransmitter that is lacking in the brains of people with Parkinson's disease, decreases as we age. Thus, if someone who is seventy-two years old is producing half as much dopamine as the average seventy-two year old, because half of their dopamine-producing cells have died and they have fewer dopamine receptors than they did at the age of sixty, which is a result of the normal aging process, they will probably show signs of moderate Parkinson's disease. This does not mean that everyone will develop Parkinson's disease as they get older. It is likely a combination of mildly reduced brain function, which is part of the normal aging process, and severe loss of dopamine-producing cells, which is part of the disease process, that results in Parkinson's disease. At this time, no one knows what other factors contribute to the risk of developing Parkinson's disease as one ages.

LIFESTYLE FACTORS THAT MAY REDUCE THE RISK OF DEVELOPING PARKINSON'S DISEASE

Not only are there factors that increase the likelihood of developing Parkinson's disease, but there are also factors that reduce the likelihood of developing Parkinson's disease as well. Current research suggests that cigarette smoking and coffee consumption may be two factors that protect against the likelihood of developing Parkinson's disease.

Several large studies have identified caffeine consumption and smoking as possible protective factors against Parkinson's disease. In a study of approximately 14,000 residents of a retirement community in southern California, Parkinson's disease was found to be significantly less common among coffee drinkers and smokers (Paganini-Hill 2001). These findings in humans have been supported by the results of studies in rodents. Caffeine has been shown to have a beneficial effect on dopamine signaling in the brain. Nicotine, the addictive component of cigarettes, also appeared to promote the effects of dopamine in the brain. These data are not meant to encourage the reader to smoke cigarettes or increase caffeine consumption. There is no evidence to support the notion that someone diagnosed with Parkinson's disease would benefit from cigarette smoking. There is certainly no evidence to support the notion that cigarette smoking or coffee consumption will prevent the development of Parkinson's disease. In contrast, there is ample evidence that smoking increases the risk of lung cancer, heart disease, and other medical conditions. Although the studies of the relationship between nicotine, caffeine, and Parkinson's disease are intriguing, this information does not support the notion that smoking or excessive caffeine consumption will reduce one's risk of developing Parkinson's disease.

4

The Treatment of Parkinson's Disease

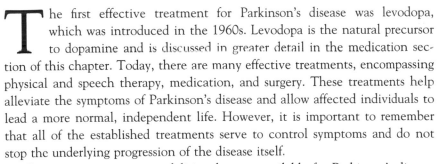

T he first effective treatment for Parkinson's disease was levodopa, which was introduced in the 1960s. Levodopa is the natural precursor to dopamine and is discussed in greater detail in the medication section of this chapter. Today, there are many effective treatments, encompassing physical and speech therapy, medication, and surgery. These treatments help alleviate the symptoms of Parkinson's disease and allow affected individuals to lead a more normal, independent life. However, it is important to remember that all of the established treatments serve to control symptoms and do not stop the underlying progression of the disease itself.

The current treatment modalities that are available for Parkinson's disease fall into one of five major categories: physical therapy, occupational therapy, speech therapy, medical treatment, and surgical treatment. Physical therapy focuses on mobility and safety in the home, workplace, and community. The therapies are designed to improve a person's motor function and strength and to maintain an adequate range of motion in the joints. Occupational therapy focuses on the use of adaptive equipment and is designed to maintain an individual's ability to live and work independently. Speech therapy focuses on communication and is designed to facilitate one's ability to interact with others.

In addition to gaining physically and improving one's communication skills from the various therapies, a person who is involved in treatment also gains psychologically by experiencing a measure of control over the symptoms of the disease. Although Parkinson's disease causes most people to become increasingly slow in their movements and muted in their speech, therapy does produce some improvements in motor and speech abilities.

PHYSICAL THERAPY

As discussed in previous chapters, Parkinson's disease is progressive. This means that the symptoms worsen over time. Because physical therapy improves motor skills, people with Parkinson's disease can benefit from undergoing physical therapy periodically, throughout the course of their illness.

Physical therapists are licensed healthcare professionals who teach a variety of strategies for coping with impairments or disabilities. These strategies help people move more easily and safely, allowing them to retain their independence. Medical centers that have a clinic specializing in Parkinson's disease usually employ physical therapists that specialize in treating their patients. The advantage of working with these physical therapists is that they are very knowledgeable about Parkinson's disease and are experienced in how the symptoms are affected by medication and other treatments. For people who live at a considerable distance from a Parkinson's disease center, it may be helpful to arrange for one comprehensive evaluation at such a center. The neurologist and the physical therapist at the center, among others, can outline a treatment plan to be followed by a doctor and therapist who live closer to one's home.

Ideally, physical therapy should include sessions in which the therapist works with the patient in his or her home and community. Particular emphasis should be placed on improving mobility in the bathroom and kitchen to avoid the risk of injury. Within the home, the bathroom is considered to be the most dangerous room. This is because the bathroom has many smooth surfaces, such as the floor of the tub and shower stall as well as the floor of the entire room, that are especially slippery when wet. The risk of falling and becoming immobile as a result of a hip fracture or broken bone is greatest in the bathroom.

Around the neighborhood, emphasis should be on safety at street crossings (including negotiating curbs) and on getting in and out of cars and buses. For someone with Parkinson's disease, it is difficult to stand when seated in a low-lying position, such as on a sofa or inside a car. To get out of a car more easily, for example, it can help to use two canes, one in either hand, for leverage.

A physical therapist will teach someone how to use both canes and get out of a car safely. In the home, sitting on chairs with armrests will help to make it easier to stand up. A person with Parkinson's disease can push up, using the armrests for leverage, to stand safely and easily.

Physical therapists can also make recommendations that help improve walking and reduce the chance of falling. People with Parkinson's disease have a tendency to take small, shuffling steps and to have difficulty stopping. A strategy to avoid these problems is to consciously think about both taking longer strides and putting the entire foot down with each step. For example, while walking down a hallway, one concentrates and says to oneself "put the heel down first, then the toe." It can also be helpful to take frequent breaks during a long walk. The rest periods are not needed as a result of fatigue, but rather, they seem to help "reset" the brain so that one's gait becomes normal again. Thus, when a person with Parkinson's disease stops, takes a short rest, and then resumes walking, the size of the initial steps can become quite normal.

Another trick for improving gait is to use visual cues to keep the size of each footstep normal and to prevent them from becoming smaller the longer one walks. Place strips of masking tape on the floor, for example, at a comfortable distance apart for a person's age, weight, and sex. Many people with Parkinson's disease find that this simple visual cue helps them walk more normally. Although it is not practical to use masking tape outside of the home, it can be quite useful in long hallways within one's house.

Fall prevention is one of the most important goals of physical therapy. More than 35 percent of people with advanced Parkinson's disease experience at least one fall. Injuries tend to be minor cuts and bruises, but about 18 percent of falls result in the fracture of one or more bones. A common symptom of Parkinson's disease that can result in falls is episodes of frozen gait.

Frozen gait refers to an episode in which the feet seem to be stuck to the floor. Despite wanting to move, a person cannot take a step and move forward. Each episode usually lasts for ten to thirty seconds. These episodes are dangerous because they may occur suddenly, without warning, and may result in a fall. Although freezing episodes can occur at any time, they are most likely to occur when someone with Parkinson's disease is negotiating a turn. Episodes of frozen gait typically begin eight to ten years after someone is diagnosed with Parkinson's disease. Some people who are prone to freezing episodes and falls find that a cane or walker helps to stay upright. Physical therapists teach several strategies that are quite useful in overcoming these episodes. Here are some examples of techniques that can be used: visualize stepping over an imaginary target or line on the floor, look ahead and focus on a distant point rather than on the floor directly under foot, count in a rhythmic cadence, and march in place. One or all of these strategies, depending on the individual, can help resume the process of taking steps and "break" the freezing episode. Episodes of freezing tend to occur when medications are wearing off and the next dose is due. This emphasizes the importance of timing physical activity and medications to minimize the risk of injury. It is best to schedule physical activity, as much as possible, to coincide with the first one to three hours after a dose of medication.

OCCUPATIONAL THERAPY

Occupational therapy focuses on helping people maintain their function despite their limitations. Occupational therapy addresses activities of daily living, such as bathing, dressing, shaving, applying makeup, eating, and writing. We tend to take these activities for granted until we can no longer perform them easily.

Occupational therapists make recommendations for adaptive equipment and for establishing new routines that will allow for continued independence at home and work. One example of adaptive equipment is the long-handled shoehorn. The handle is long enough that someone can sit in a chair and put their shoes on without having to lean forward. Because people with Parkinson's disease have difficulty maintaining their balance, using a long-handled shoehorn eliminates the need to bend forward and down while putting on shoes, thus eliminating the risk of falling while performing this basic task.

Another example of adaptive equipment is a shower bench. A shower bench is a plastic, nonskid bench that is placed in the bathtub or shower stall. It allows the user to sit while washing one's self, thereby reducing the risk of slipping and falling. The combination of slippery, hard surfaces and water make the bathtub or shower stall potentially hazardous for anyone but particularly for someone with Parkinson's disease. A shower bench is a simple tool that gives someone with Parkinson's disease the ability to continue to bathe themselves, in their own home, in a safe manner.

The tremor associated with Parkinson's disease can make it difficult to eat a bowl of soup or hold a cup of coffee. To minimize the tremor and ease any difficulty with eating, occupational therapists may recommend using weighted eating utensils. Many different types of modified eating utensils are available, and so it is important for someone with Parkinson's disease to go over their difficulties and their typical diet with an occupational therapist so that they get the utensils that will help them the most.

Micrographia, the small cramped handwriting that is a symptom of Parkinson's disease, can be quite frustrating and disabling to the person affected.

Unfortunately, the medications that are used to treat Parkinson's disease, which improve gait and minimize resting tremor, have little effect on hand-writing. However, difficulty with handwriting can be compensated for by the use of a computer. Typing on a keyboard can be much easier than writing with a pen or pencil. Also, a wide variety of modified keyboards are available, with wider keys for each letter and greater space between the keys such that it is easier for someone with Parkinson's disease to use them.

In summary, occupational therapy treatments that are specific for those with Parkinson's disease include a home exercise program for the arms to maintain strength and promote flexibility, the establishment of a routine for activities of daily living (bathing, dressing, the application of makeup) that is timed to coincide with the onset of medication and that includes rest periods to compensate for fatigue, and the use of adaptive equipment.

A Typical Day Improved by a Physical or Occupational Therapist

So what do physical and occupational therapy sessions really do for people with Parkinson's disease? Let us go through a typical day in the life of a person with Parkinson's disease, highlighting activities that have been or can be improved with physical and occupational therapy.

Jose is a fifty-year-old stockbroker who lives in Connecticut and works in New York City. Jose lives alone and was diagnosed with Parkinson's disease three years ago when he was experiencing a tremor in his right hand whenever he laid it down on a desk or the arm of a chair. He takes medication, to control the tremor, four times a day. Jose typically wakes up at 5:30 A.M. The medi-cation he takes at bedtime works through the night, so he is only a little stiff and slow in the morning. Once he wakes up, Jose begins to review in his mind the movements he must perform to get out of bed without falling or feeling light headed. Then Jose sits up, swings his legs over the side of the bed, and counts to twenty. He then puts his feet down and, using his arms, pushes himself up into a standing position. As he walks across the bedroom to the bathroom, Jose reminds himself to place first his heel firmly on the floor, followed by the ball of his foot, and then his toes.

In the bathroom, Jose has no difficulty using the toilet and taking a shower, thanks to assistive devices that were installed last year that make it easier to get up from the toilet. Jose installed a raised toilet seat with armrests. He also had a grab bar installed in the shower and uses a nonslip bath mat on the tub floor. Very importantly, he does not rely on a towel bar to hold him up should he slip in the shower. A towel bar has only enough strength to hold the weight of a few towels. The grab bar Jose installed is textured, drilled securely into the wall studs, and designed specifically to hold the weight of an adult. Once bathed and dressed, Jose heads to the kitchen for a full breakfast and his morning dose of medication.

Because Jose has trouble with fine motor movement, he uses a rocker knife and other adaptive kitchen utensils to prepare and eat a meal of fruit, egg-white omelet, and coffee. Jose learned about and ordered this equipment with the assistance of his occupational therapist. After breakfast, Jose drives to the train station and catches the train to Manhattan. Jose and his neurologist have timed his morning medication dose so that it kicks in as his train reaches his destination, Grand Central Station. Jose gets off the train and walks to work, focusing on taking big, complete steps. He gets to the office in time for the opening bell of the stock market and gets to work.

By the end of the workday, Jose is exhausted. His tremor is more pronounced and his ability to use a computer keyboard is markedly worse than it had been in the morning. Fortunately, Jose has an office with a couch and can take a nap. Before the nap, he takes a dose of medication so he can easily walk back to the train station.

Jose is aggressive in the treatment of his symptoms of Parkinson's disease. He maintains an active and independent lifestyle. Below is another case, of Elena, a woman who is less aggressive in her philosophy about illness and more sedentary than Jose. Nevertheless, Elena obtained benefit and relief from some of her Parkinson's symptoms by using multiple types of treatment.

Elena is seventy-four and was diagnosed with Parkinson's disease five years ago. She has been on the same medication regimen since she was first diagnosed and has not researched the disease or asked many questions of her doctor. She takes the medication as prescribed and does not want to "bother" her doctor with too many questions. She worries that her doctor will think that she is complaining about the care that she receives. Elena's daughter, Joy, has noticed that her mother is becoming slower and slower in her movements and that her voice is more breathy. It is difficult to understand her mother when they are talking on the telephone. Joy has also witnessed a few near-falls that have her worried that her mom could fall and break a bone. Out of concern, Joy made an appointment for her mom with a doctor at the Parkinson's disease clinic at a nearby medical center.

Joy accompanied her mom to the appointment and told the neurologist, Dr. Lee, about the changes she noticed in her mom's mobility and overall health. Based on the information provided by Elena and Joy and the exam itself, Dr. Lee changed Elena's medication regimen.

Dr. Lee also arranged for physical therapy sessions with a therapist who works extensively with people who have Parkinson's disease. In addition, Dr. Lee had the visiting nurse assess Elena's home to ensure that she was safe and to determine whether grab bars should be put in the tub or area rugs removed. Thus, by optimizing medications and taking advantage of the services provided by a multidisciplinary treatment team, Elena improved her mobility and continued to live in her own home.

SPEECH THERAPY

Speech-language therapists work with people who have any of a variety of disorders that affect the ability to make the sounds of speech clearly or at all. The therapists concentrate on the mechanics of speech that are needed to produce the sounds that we use, including the movement of a person's tongue, lips, cheeks, and throat. They also focus on aspects of breathing that are important for creating clear speech. Because the muscles that create clear speech are also involved in chewing and swallowing food, people with speech difficulty frequently also have eating difficulties. Speech therapists also work with people who have difficulty eating and swallowing because of problems with the movement of their mouth. People with Parkinson's disease typically have trouble with both producing clear speech and swallowing safely.

Hypophonia is one example of a speech disorder that is found in people with Parkinson's disease. Hypophonia refers to a reduction in the loudness of the voice. Typically, hypophonia develops within the first five years of the onset of Parkinson's disease. In this early stage of Parkinson's disease, a person's voice is hypophonic but their pronunciation is relatively clear. Thus, speech therapy consists of maneuvers to improve the working of a person's natural vocal apparatus. These maneuvers do help patients make improvements in the intelligibility and loudness of their speech and their rate of speaking.

A program called the Lee Silverman Voice Treatment (LSVT) program has been shown to be effective in improving both the volume and speech of patients in the early stages of Parkinson's disease (Ramig et al. 2001). The LSVT program is a compensatory maneuver that focuses on speaking in a louder voice. The LSVT program consists of an intensive schedule of sixteen individual speech sessions that take place over a one month period. The program focuses on optimizing sounds low in the throat. Studies have shown that 90 percent of patients improve after LSVT and that, of these, 80 percent maintain improvement in their voice for six to twelve months.

In the later stages of Parkinson's disease, the ability to speak clearly may become significantly impaired. This typically develops ten to twenty years after the disease is diagnosed. At this stage, someone with Parkinson's disease may find it difficult to consistently maintain an adequate level of loudness in the voice. The voice may be so soft that it is extremely difficult, if not impossible, to do anything more complicated than answer "yes" or "no" to simple questions. As one can imagine, this is frustrating for the person with Parkinson's disease, whose mind is intact but who cannot have even casual conversations with others. It is important to remember that speech therapy can be enormously helpful at this stage of the disease. A speech therapist can help improve communication by teaching the use of aids such as an easy-to-use message board or a voice amplification system. Voice amplification systems consist of a lightweight speaker that is attached at the waist with a belt and a lightweight microphone that rests unobtrusively around the neck. These amplification systems make the voice louder, thus making communication easier.

The goal of speech therapy in Parkinson's disease is to improve and stabilize voice quality for a period of time. The benefits of speech therapy do not end there, because a variety of assistive devices can also be used to make communication easier as the symptoms of Parkinson's disease progress. Speech therapy is not a once-in-a-lifetime treatment, and most people find that repeated therapy over the years does have some benefit in improving the quality of their voice.

Because the muscles that control speech are also involved in swallowing, the appearance of hypophonia in someone with Parkinson's disease also indicates that some element of dysphagia is present. Dysphagia refers to difficulty swallowing, and its severity is usually proportional to the decline in the loudness of someone's speech. Dysphagia can be assessed using an x-ray study, ordered by a physician. The study is referred to as a barium swallow. The test requires that a patient drink and swallow a radio-opaque liquid. While the patient is drinking and swallowing the liquid, an x-ray technician obtains images of the mouth and throat. The images follow the route of the liquid within the body. If there is no dysphagia, the liquid flows easily from the tip of the tongue to the back of the throat, down the esophagus, and into the stomach. If dysphagia is present, the liquid may sit on the tongue for a longer period than is normal. Upon reaching the back of the throat, some of the liquid may then enter the trachea and reach the lungs. If the radio-opaque dye enters the lungs, it is likely that food can enter the lungs as well. The term "aspiration" refers to the ingestion of food particles into the lungs. In a person with Parkinson's disease, it is more difficult to cough up the food or other substance that has gone into the lungs by mistake. The result is that this piece of food will block an airway and bacteria will now be able to grow behind the food, resulting in pneumonia. A speech therapist can teach specific exercises and techniques that will improve swallowing in a person with Parkinson's disease who has dysphagia.

Jennifer is fifty-nine years old and has a son, Josh, who is twenty years old. Jennifer was diagnosed with Parkinson's disease two years ago, and her symptoms are well controlled with medication. Josh goes to college in Chicago, 1,000 miles away from home. Josh calls his mom faithfully every Sunday and does get worried about her disease and how she is coping because she lives alone and he doesn't see her that often.

In the last year, Josh has noticed that it is harder to understand his mom when they talk on the telephone. At first, Jennifer ignored his comments about this, assuming that he just had his stereo on too loud whenever they talked. However, friends at work began to ask Jennifer to speak up, because they had trouble understanding her, too. Jennifer talked to her primary care doctor about it. Her primary care doctor thought that the speech changes were related to the Parkinson's disease and suggested that she see her neurologist. The neurologist agreed that the speech changes were related to the Parkinson's disease and referred her for LSVT with a speech therapist. Just to be sure, he also ordered a barium swallow x-ray study to confirm that she was swallowing her food properly. Jennifer found that she was able to speak more loudly and clearly, both at work and when on the phone, after she underwent intensive speech therapy. Fortunately, there was no evidence of dysphagia on the x-ray study, so she can continue to eat whatever she would like without worrying about how to chew or swallow.

MEDICAL TREATMENT

Medical treatment refers to the use of medication to relieve the symptoms of Parkinson's disease. There are a variety of medications available to treat the symptoms of Parkinson's disease (see Table 4.1). To date, there are no medications to stop the progression of Parkinson's disease. The majority of patients use a combination of medications to relieve their symptoms. Typically, patients are on one or, at most, two medications to relieve their symptoms for the first three to five years after they are diagnosed with Parkinson's disease. In this early stage, medication is taken three times a day. However, as the disease progresses, more medications are needed to provide greater relief of symptoms and allow people to live independently. As the disease progresses, people with Parkinson's disease find that they need to take three or more different medicines five or six times a day.

Table 4.1.
Medications Used in the Treatment of Parkinson's Disease

Drug class	Generic name	Brand name
Anticholinergic	benztropine	Cogentin
	trihexyphenidyl	Artane
Antiviral	amantadine	Symmetrel
Dopamine replacement	carbidopa/levodopa	Sinemet
Dopamine agonists	bromocriptine	Parlodel
	ropinirole	Requip
	pramipexole	Mirapex
	rotigotine	Neupro
MAO-B inhibitor	selegiline	Deprenyl
	rasagiline	Azilect
COMT inhibitor	entacapone	Comtan
	tolcapone	Tasmar
Combination dopamine replacement + COMT inhibitor	carbidopa/levodopa + entacapone	Stalevo

The decision about when to start taking medication is based on a patient's degree of disability and discomfort. Neurologists prescribe these medications based on symptoms and the individual's response to various dosages. The goal of medical treatment is to help the patient function independently for as long as possible. Six classes of drugs are available to help accomplish this goal: anticholinergic agents, antiviral drug, dopamine replacement agents, dopamine agonists, inhibitors of the enzyme monoamine oxidase B (MAO-B), and inhibitors of the enzyme catechol-*o*-methyl transferase (COMT). Each medication has a generic name, which is listed first in this book, and a brand name, which is listed in parentheses after the generic name.

Brand-Name versus Generic Drugs

When a pharmaceutical company develops a new drug, the company applies to a government patent office for a patent. A patent gives the company exclusive rights to produce and sell the drug without competition from other companies. In most countries, the life of a patent is twenty years from registration. The intention of a patent is to allow a company to recoup its investment in developing a drug and make a profit from selling the drug. The pharmaceutical company also applies to the national trademark office to obtain permission for the exclusive use of a particular name. This name is the brand name of the particular drug and is registered to the company, thus becoming the property of that company. After a patent expires, other pharmaceutical companies may manufacture and sell the original drug as a generic drug. The generic drug must contain the same medicinal ingredient(s) as the brand-name version. Companies that make generic drugs do not have to invest the millions of dollars that were required to develop and bring a specific drug to market. As a result, the makers of generic drugs can charge a significantly lower price for the same medication.

Anticholinergic Agents

Anticholinergic agents are the oldest class of medications used for the treatment of Parkinson's disease. Two of the most widely available agents are trihexyphenidyl (Artane) and benztropine (Cogentin). They work by blocking the effects of a neurotransmitter called acetylcholine and are most effective in reducing rest tremor and rigidity. However, they have side effects that typically limit their use. The side effects include dry mouth, constipation, urinary retention, blurred vision, confusion, and difficulty with concentration. With the development and availability of more effective drugs that also have fewer side effects, the use of anticholinergic agents in the treatment of Parkinson's disease has declined dramatically. In the United States, these medications are not commonly used for the treatment of Parkinson's disease. However, in other parts of the world where people do not have the funds to purchase newer, more effective medications, these medicines are still used.

Antiviral Agent

Amantadine (Symmetrel) is also used to treat Parkinson's disease. Amantadine is classified as an antiviral drug that is used to prevent and treat respiratory infections caused by the influenza A virus. The way in which amantadine works in people with Parkinson's disease is not fully understood. However, amantadine is thought to work by augmenting the release of dopamine from those neurons that are still healthy and producing dopamine. Amantadine produces limited improvement in bradykinesia (slow movement), rigidity, and rest tremor. Amantadine is more effective in controlling the dyskinesias that can develop later in the course of Parkinson's disease. Dyskinesias are discussed in greater detail in Chapter 5. Possible side effects of amantadine include lower extremity edema (swelling caused by accumulation of fluid), confusion, and hallucinations. In particular, it is the confusion that limits the use of amantadine.

Dopamine Replacement

Dopamine replacement is the cornerstone of therapy for Parkinson's disease. Patients take a drug called levodopa rather than dopamine. Levodopa is the natural precursor to dopamine and is given in combination with another medication called carbidopa. Carbidopa helps the levodopa enter the brain by blocking the breakdown of levodopa in the bloodstream, before its entry into the brain itself. Once levodopa enters the brain, it is converted to dopamine.

Levodopa is most effective in reducing tremor, rigidity, and bradykinesia. The most common side effects, seen with the onset of treatment, are nausea and abdominal cramping. These side effects typically only last for a few weeks, at the most. In most people, starting the medication at a very low dose and increasing it slowly helps to minimize, if not eliminate, the experience of side effects. Once the body becomes used to the levodopa, these side effects disappear. Long-term treatment with levodopa or the dopamine agonists is associated with two potential types of complications: hourly fluctuations in motor state and dyskinesias. It is not clear whether these complications are the result of the medications, the progression of the underlying disease, or some complex interaction between these two factors. These and other long-term complications of Parkinson's disease are discussed in greater detail in Chapter 5.

Dopamine Agonists

An agonist is a drug that binds to and activates a receptor on a cell, leading to changes within that cell. Dopamine agonists work by directly stimulating dopamine receptors on brain cells. Dopamine agonists fool the brain into thinking that there is more dopamine present than there really is. Several dopamine agonists are available and can be given orally or through a skin patch. They can be used alone or in combination with levodopa therapy. There is limited evidence that suggests that, by using dopamine agonists first and by avoiding the use of levodopa during the first two years of treatment, there may be less risk of developing dyskinesias later in the course of the disease. However, this possible benefit to the use of the newer dopamine agonists has not been conclusively demonstrated in long-term clinical trials.

Bromocriptine (Parlodel) is one of the first dopamine agonist medications that was developed and became available for patient use. Bromocriptine is less specific in its actions than the newer generation of dopamine agonists. The newer dopamine agonists pramipexole (Mirapex) and ropinirole (Requip) are more specific in their actions and thus, in theory, are less likely to cause side effects. Compared with levodopa, both the new and old dopamine agonists cause a lower frequency of dyskinesias and a higher frequency of confusion and hallucinations. To minimize the risk of intolerable side effects, it is best for a patient to start with a small dose of medication taken only once a day, in the morning or afternoon, and then slowly increase the total daily dosage.

Gradually, the medication dose is increased. All three of these drugs, bromocriptine, pramipexole, and ropinirole, are taken in tablet form. Bromocriptine tablets should be taken twice a day. Both pramipexole and ropinirole tablets should be taken three times a day. Because all three medications tend to cause confusion, particularly at night, it is important to slowly increase the total daily dose, over several weeks, to minimize the chance that the person taking the medication will develop side effects. In general, when medications are started at a low dose and increased slowly, a person can tolerate high doses without difficulty. Problems arise when a medication is started at a relatively high dose or the total daily dose is increased too quickly.

A relatively new dopamine agonist, known as rotigotine (Neupro), is available in a patch formulation. The patch is applied to the skin, and the medication is absorbed at a relatively steady rate through the skin and then enters the bloodstream. This drug delivery system is thought to result in more steady-state blood levels of a particular drug when compared with taking the same medication orally. With oral ingestion of medication, blood levels of a particular drug peak approximately one hour after the pill is swallowed and then steadily decline until the next pill is taken. Thus, the theory is that, if a medication is delivered at a steady rate throughout the day, this is a better mimic of what the body would normally do if it were healthy. However, no one knows whether delivering a medication via patch rather than via a tablet will affect the long-term, progressive course of Parkinson's disease. In fact, it is not clear whether the patch formulation of a dopamine agonist provides better control of Parkinson's disease symptoms than the oral formulation.

MAO-B Inhibitors of Dopamine Metabolism

Inhibitors of dopamine metabolism are also used to treat Parkinson's disease. Metabolism occurs within the body and encompasses all the steps involved in the breakdown of naturally occurring chemicals or exogenously administered medications. Thus, agents that inhibit the metabolism of dopamine will allow the dopamine to remain in its active state for a longer period. Selegiline (Deprenyl) is an inhibitor of dopamine metabolism. It inhibits the enzyme MAO-B, which acts in the central nervous system by breaking down dopamine. Common side effects include dry mouth and dizziness. A newer medication, rasagiline (Azilect), is also an inhibitor of MAO-B, thus allowing dopamine to remain active for a longer period. It is not clear whether there are significant differences between these two medications, although it is clear that medications that work by inhibiting MAO-B are helpful in the treatment of Parkinson's disease.

COMT Inhibitors of Dopamine Metabolism

Entacapone (Comtan) is another inhibitor of dopamine metabolism. Entacapone inhibits the activity of the enzyme known as COMT. COMT is an enzyme that breaks down levodopa in the blood before it gets to the brain. Entacapone is taken in conjunction with a tablet of carbidopa/levodopa and acts to increase the amount of levodopa that reaches the brain. The most common side effects of entacapone are abdominal pain and fatigue. The benefits of entacapone treatment include a reduction in total daily levodopa dose, an improvement in the length of time of optimal mobility, and a reduction in the number of times during the day that a person has to take medication.

A recently released medication is a combination pill of entacapone with carbidopa and levodopa. The brand name of this drug is Stalevo. The advantage to this combination pill is that it reduces the number of tablets a person has to take on a daily basis. Common side effects of Stalevo include nausea and headache.

Tolcapone (Tasmar) is another inhibitor of COMT. Similar to entacapone, tolcapone is taken in conjunction with a tablet of carbidopa/levodopa and acts to increase the amount of levodopa that reaches the brain. A rare, but fatal, risk from taking tolcapone is acute liver failure. Because of this risk, the use of tolcapone is typically limited to people who either cannot tolerate or do not derive benefits from other medications for their Parkinson's disease. People who are on tolcapone also get frequent blood tests to ensure that their liver is not being damaged by the medication.

As you can see, there are many choices for the medical treatment of the symptoms of Parkinson's disease. These medications are effective in controlling the symptoms of Parkinson's disease and allowing people to continue to lead independent lives. However, every medication has side effects. It is important to work closely with a neurologist to devise an optimal treatment plan. It is also important to remember that there is no treatment that slows the progression of Parkinson's disease.

SURGICAL TREATMENT

Although many medications are available for treating early and moderately advanced Parkinson's disease, their use is limited in more advanced cases. This is when surgery can be useful. Several surgical procedures are either currently available or being actively studied in research laboratories. Information about them will continue to grow over the next several years.

Surgical approaches for treating advanced Parkinson's disease fall into one of five categories: restorative (cell transplantation), maintenance (use of growth factors), ablative (thalamotomy or pallidotomy), gene therapy, and electrophysiological (deep brain stimulation [DBS]).

Restorative Surgery

Cell transplantation is still an experimental approach in the treatment of Parkinson's disease. The goal is to replace the lost dopamine-producing brain neurons. At this time, four different sources of dopamine-producing cells are being studied. Essentially, these four possible sources of dopamine cells can be classified into one of two categories: immature human cells and cells from other animals.

Immature human cells have the capacity to develop into one of the many different types of cells found in the body. The process whereby an immature cell develops into a fully formed, adult cell is referred to as differentiation. As a human fetus develops, immature cells differentiate into liver cells, heart cells, and brain cells, among others. Within each of these organs, cells in different regions develop in distinct patterns and serve unique functions. As a result, once an immature human cell has differentiated into a liver cell, for example, it cannot revert back to its original form and become any other type of cell. The key to research in this area is to first identify and harvest cells when they are truly immature, before they have begun on the path of differentiation. The next, equally important, step is to develop the methods by which these cells can be coaxed along into developing as mature dopamine-producing brain cells. The goal is to promote their differentiation into dopamine neurons and then implant them into the brain. This is an area of active research, in which significant advances are being made on a regular basis.

Human Fetal Neuronal Cells

In animal models of Parkinson's disease, transplants of fetal brain cells have been shown to work reasonably well. The outcome in humans, however, is not so encouraging. In a recent study in which human embryonic dopamine neurons were transplanted into the brains of patients with severe Parkinson's disease, there was no significant, long-term improvement in symptoms. One critical issue, which no one understands, is how to ensure that the implanted cells form the proper connection with other cells in the brain.

Human Adult Precursor Cells

Some people think that, within an adult human brain, there are some undifferentiated cells. The theory is that, once identified, these cells can be isolated and manipulated, in a laboratory, to develop into dopamine-producing cells that can then be reimplanted in the human brain. Because such a technique would not involve the use of fetal tissue, which arouses significant controversy, many people hope that this will be an equally useful approach. However, no one has shown that neuronal precursors exist in the adult human brain.

Previous work along these lines in patients with Parkinson's disease used cells not from the brain but from the adult adrenal gland. The adrenal gland is an organ that sits on top of the kidney. Some cells within the adrenal gland produce dopamine. The adrenal dopamine cells were isolated and then inserted into the brains of some patients with Parkinson's disease. Unfortunately, the results were disappointing.

Embryonic Stem Cells

Embryonic stem (ES) cells are initially obtained from a developing human embryo about four to seven days after an egg is fertilized. ES cells are pluripotent, meaning that they can develop into any number of the specialized types of cells of the human body. The removed ES cells are grown in the laboratory where they increase in number and can be induced to change their characteristics, such that they develop into one of many of the mature cells found in an adult.

The hope is that ES cells can be used to treat a variety of diseases, including Parkinson's disease, Alzheimer's disease, and diabetes. Although the availability of limited federal and private funds is expected to accelerate the rate of research, there is considerable work to do before ES cell-based therapies are ready to be used in humans, even experimentally.

For Parkinson's disease, intensive research programs are underway to determine how to stimulate ES cells into becoming dopamine-producing cells that could then be transplanted into the human brain. The ES cells would provide an unlimited supply of the highly specialized, dopamine-producing neurons. However, the secrets of how to change ES cells into dopamine-producing neurons and then to safely insert them among other brain cells has yet to be discovered.

A recent study, done in a monkey model of Parkinson's disease, illustrates how difficult this work can be (Redmond et al. 2007). Monkeys were treated with MPTP, the toxin that targets and destroys dopamine neurons that was discussed in Chapter 1. The monkeys that had the most severe symptoms of Parkinson's disease (bradykinesia, tremor, and freezing episodes) were selected for surgery. Some of these monkeys received stem cells and some underwent surgery without receiving any stem cells. In the first four months after the surgery, the monkeys that received the stem cells displayed a marked improvement in their symptoms. Unfortunately, the improvements wore off after four months, and those monkeys that received the stem cells appeared to be no different from those monkeys that underwent surgery and did not receive the stem cells. When the brains from those monkeys were studied under a microscope, the researchers were surprised to discover that most of the injected stem cells had not gone on to produce dopamine.

Xenotransplantation

Xenotransplantation refers to the transfer of nonhuman tissue into the human body. A significant risk of xenotransplantation is that animal viruses or bacteria may be introduced into humans. A recent study to evaluate the safety of and potential benefit from the transplantation of pig embryonic brain cells into twelve people with Parkinson's disease has been reported. One year after the surgery, there was no evidence of infection by a pig virus in the recipients. However, there was not a significant improvement in the symptoms of Parkinson's disease either. These results indicate that xenotransplantation may be safe in humans. However, there is no evidence that the cells were helpful within the first year of surgery. There is still no data regarding its safety and effectiveness over five, ten, or more years after the surgery. Research to refine the techniques used in xenotransplantation, with an emphasis on minimizing the risk of introducing animal viruses into humans, continues.

Maintenance Therapy

An alternative approach is to deliver growth factors to the brain that would promote the survival of those dopamine-producing neurons that are still alive. One of the compounds under study is called glial cell-line-derived neurotrophic factor (GDNF). During fetal brain development, GDNF is needed for the proper development of dopamine-producing neurons. Thus, it is reasonable to think that giving GDNF to someone whose dopamine neurons are dying may help the cells survive. GDNF was first studied in a rat model of Parkinson's disease, in which the results were promising. A small-scale human trial was then initiated. However, a preliminary analysis that was done early in the course of treatment with GDNF did not find a significant improvement in Parkinson's symptoms in those who took GDNF. In addition, simultaneous work was being conducted with GDNF in monkeys. Several monkeys that were treated with GDNF developed damage in their cerebellum. The cerebellum is the part of the brain that controls coordination. You may wonder why this complication was not seen in the rats that were treated with GDNF. The brain of a rat is very different from a human brain. In fact, it is only non-human primates, such as monkeys, who display a complex brain organization similar to that of humans. This is why drugs that are active in the brain are best tested in monkeys as well as rodents. As a result of the complications found when monkeys were treated with GDNF, the human clinical trials were stopped. Although the result is disappointing, this is a good example of the importance of doing extensive research in multiple different animal models of a particular disease rather than simply directly testing compounds in humans. To develop safe and effective treatments for humans, it is essential to first test potential medicines in other animals.

Gene Therapy

Gene therapy is a technique whereby a specific gene is introduced into the human body. The goal is to have that gene produce its specific protein, which is either not present at all or present at low levels, in a particular organ of the body. As we discussed in Chapter 3, very few cases of Parkinson's disease are caused by an inherited mutation in one's DNA. Thus, trying to administer a normal copy of a gene, in which a mutation causes Parkinson's disease in only a few people, is not being pursued at this time. The consensus amongst scientists, physicians, and those who help to establish healthcare policy is that it makes more sense to fund research programs that are likely to benefit a larger number of people with Parkinson's disease.

There is, however, a way in which gene therapy could help many people with Parkinson's disease. If a gene could be administered that helps to alleviate the symptoms of Parkinson's disease, regardless of how a person developed the disease, then this gene could be used in the same way that oral medications are used today. With this in mind, gene therapy is being used to introduce many copies of the gene that produces a neurotransmitter called GABA (also called 4-aminobutyrate) into the subthalamic nucleus. The subthalamic nucleus is a specific region of the brain. It is thought that some of the symptoms of Parkinson's disease are caused by the overactivity of cells within the subthalamic nucleus. The neurotransmitter GABA serves to "calm" brain cells. The goal of this study is to introduce many copies of the gene that directs the production of GABA, resulting in high levels of the neurotransmitter GABA in the subthalamic nucleus. The hypothesis is that, by increasing the levels of GABA, the brain cells in the subthalamic nucleus will become less active, resulting in greater control over the symptoms of Parkinson's disease.

A small number of patients, who all knew that they were getting the gene for GABA, participated in a clinical trial. Preliminary results, indicating that the treatment is safe and may be helpful in controlling their symptoms, were announced just before the publication of this book. Although these data are potentially very exciting, it is important to be cautious and thoughtful in reviewing the results and thinking about the meaning of these results. First, all the patients and all the physicians evaluating the patients knew that they were getting the gene for GABA. Ideally, neither the patients nor the evaluating doctors should know who truly received the treatment under study and who received an inactive, placebo treatment. The reason for this is that it is better if the doctors who evaluate the results of a treatment are not biased by their own desire to help people with a particular disease. Thus, the report of an improvement in Parkinson's symptoms in a small number of people who received the gene for GABA may have been affected by the fact that both the patients and the doctors want to see an improvement. Another concern about this study is that only twelve patients were treated. To be certain that GABA gene therapy, or any other treatment, is effective for Parkinson's disease, it must be tested in hundreds of people, of both genders and different ethnic backgrounds.

Ablative Surgery

Ablative surgical treatment is a technique that was introduced years ago for treating Parkinson's disease, before oral medications were available. It is used to destroy specific structures of the brain within the basal ganglia in which the symptoms arise. One of two distinct regions of the basal ganglia is targeted for destruction, depending on a patient's symptoms. The surgery creates damage that is irreversible.

Some patients today, whose symptoms do not respond to medication, can benefit from ablative surgery. One approach is called a pallidotomy in which a surgeon creates a lesion in a portion of the brain called the globus pallidus. The globus pallidus is a part of the brain that collects information from the body, synthesizes the information, and then sends it along to other areas in the brain. This procedure is recommended for some patients who experience bradykinesia, rigidity, tremor, and significant drug-induced dyskinesia despite optimal medical therapy.

Thalamotomy is another type of ablative surgical treatment in which the neurosurgeon makes a lesion in a specific region of the thalamus. The thalamus is a part of the brain with many functions. Some of its functions include relaying sensory information between different areas of the brain and helping to control our muscles and limbs. Thalamotomy is recommended for those with Parkinson's disease who have an asymmetric, severe, medically intractable tremor.

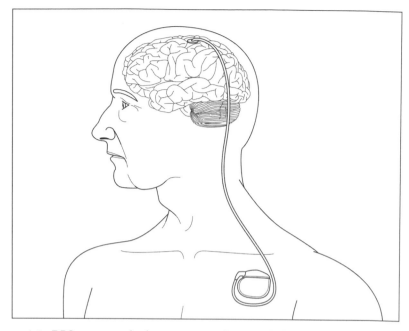

Figure 4.1. DBS consists of a battery source that rests below the collarbone and just under the skin. Electrodes from the battery are threaded into the brain, where they generate a magnetic field whose size can be adjusted by changing the settings on the battery. A neurologist makes changes to the battery settings during an office visit, using a handheld device that is placed on the skin on top of the battery. These adjustments to the battery settings are noninvasive. *Illustrated by Jeff Dixon.*

Electrophysiological Treatment

In DBS, high-frequency electrical pulses are applied via a wire or wires to one of several locations in the basal ganglia. DBS requires surgery in which a device (such as a pacemaker), for providing electrical stimulation, is placed under the skin of the chest while its wires are threaded into the subthalamic nucleus, thalamus, or globus pallidus of the brain (see Figure 4.1). The electrical stimulation is thought to block the signals that cause the disabling motor symptoms in Parkinson's disease. The extent of stimulation can be adjusted, by an experienced neurologist, using a hand-held device that is placed on the surface of the skin, just above the site where the device was placed (typically just below the collarbone).

DBS surgery is a major undertaking and requires an extensive evaluation at a Parkinson's disease center as well as thoughtful consideration by a patient and his or her family. It is important to weigh the risk and benefits of the surgery carefully. Surgical treatment for medication-resistant Parkinson's disease is an important and rapidly expanding therapeutic option. In carefully selected cases, surgical treatment can have a significant positive effect on symptoms.

Patients are given a local anesthetic and sedation, so that they will not feel any pain when the hard, bony skull is cut. However, some patient cooperation is required during the procedure, so that the patient is often drowsy but easily awakened. During the second part of the operation, when the battery is placed under the collarbone, patients are put under general anesthesia. With general anesthesia, patients are "asleep" and not aware of feeling any pain from the surgical procedure. Typically, several weeks after the surgical procedures are complete, the patient returns to the neurologist's office to have the stimulator turned on and the settings adjusted. The doctor will make adjustments to the stimulator settings that modify the strength and shape of the electric field produced within the brain. The advantage of DBS is that, once the unit is in place, the degree of electrical stimulation can be easily adjusted. Trained medical personnel use a device called a controller, which sits on the skin and communicates with the stimulator that is inside the body. With the controller, one can adjust the size and shape of the magnetic field inside the brain. The goal of this treatment is to establish an optimal magnetic field that disrupts the abnormal signals that the brain is sending. By disrupting those abnormal signals, some of the signs and symptoms of Parkinson's disease become less severe.

The advantage of the deep brain stimulator, when compared with treatment by thalamotomy or pallidotomy, is that the size of the "lesion" (i.e., the magnetic field) can be easily altered. For those who receive a thalamotomy or pallidotomy, in contrast, the lesion is fixed and permanent. The disadvantage of the deep brain stimulator is that the optimal size of the magnetic field is determined slowly, typically over the course of one year after the surgery. This requires frequent trips to the neurologist's office. However, once optimal settings are established, people are able to take less oral medication and have better mobility. Another disadvantage to treatment with the deep brain stimulator is that the battery, located under the collarbone, requires replacement once every three years, on average. Thus, in addition to undergoing one surgery within the brain, a Parkinson's patient is committing themselves to undergoing general anesthesia once every three years, for the rest of their lives. Those who receive a thalamotomy or pallidotomy do not have to undergo additional surgeries. Although the results from DBS or more traditional surgeries that create an unchangeable lesion can be striking, the risks and benefits of these procedures should be considered carefully and discussed with one's doctors extensively.

5

The Course and Complications of Parkinson's Disease

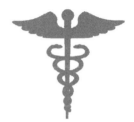

Janet Reno served as the United States Attorney General for eight years during the administration of President William Clinton. Early during her tenure, she was diagnosed with Parkinson's disease. Despite this, she continued to serve the President and the nation. As attorney general, Ms. Reno represented the United States in legal matters and gave legal advice to the President and to the heads of the various departments of the Government when so requested. Over the years, Ms. Reno frequently appeared before congressional committees. As the years passed, those in congress as well as the public noted that her arms would shake more noticeably and her speech was softer. However, Ms. Reno continued to fulfill the duties of her position without difficulty. She oversaw all legal work at the Justice Department and continued to give clear and thoughtful legal advice to the President and other members of the cabinet.

Pope John Paul II, who served as leader of the Catholic Church from 1978 until his death in 2005, had Parkinson's disease. Although no definitive information has been released by the Vatican, it was clear to those who observed him in the last ten years of his life that the pope had difficulty speaking, was visibly frail, and had difficulty walking. In 2003, a cardinal confirmed that the *pope had been diagnosed with Parkinson's disease. Despite his physical difficulties, which led him to turn over much of his weekly physical duties, such as leading mass, to a cardinal, Pope John Paul II continued to lead the church. He made decisions on theological questions that served to guide Catholics all over the world. Thus, despite physical frailty, the pope was able to serve as spiritual leader of a faith with adherents throughout the world.*

Parkinson's disease is a slowly progressive disorder. The onset of symptoms is gradual. Typically, stiffness and slowness develops over twelve to eighteen months before a person realizes that something serious is happening and seeks medical attention. The presence of a rest tremor may become obvious over a shorter period of time, typically six to twelve months, and typically pushes the person with the tremor to seek medical attention relatively quickly.

At the time of diagnosis, it is estimated that about 70 percent of the dopamine-producing cells in the brain have already died. It is clear that we have a considerable reserve in our brain, allowing for the loss of a significant amount of dopamine production, before our body exhibits any symptoms of Parkinson's disease. As discussed in Chapter 4, there is currently no treatment that prevents or slows the progressive loss of dopamine-producing neurons. It is the goal of physicians and scientists to develop a means to identify those people who are losing dopamine-producing brain cells before they display any signs of Parkinson's disease and then treat them with medications that will prevent the loss of any more brain cells. Thus, the long-term goal is to prevent people from developing Parkinson's disease. This is an area of intensive research in which new information is generated on an almost annual basis. In future editions of this and other books about Parkinson's disease, it is likely that entire chapters will be devoted to the issues of identifying those at risk for developing the disease and the use of medication to prevent additional loss of dopamine-producing cells. Unfortunately, at this time, there is no means to identify those who will develop Parkinson's disease, nor is there treatment to prevent the progression of the disease.

At first in Parkinson's disease, people typically begin to notice changes in the way they walk or feel. This usually goes on for a while before they bring it to the attention of their physician. When people discuss their symptoms with a doctor, they might talk about feeling shaky and slow, sore, or weak. Parkinson's disease can be confused with a number of other conditions so the doctor will be looking for its cardinal signs. As mentioned in Chapter 2, physicians use the term "cardinal signs" to describe features that are most common in people with a given disease. In Parkinson's disease, these signs are caused by the loss of cells that produce dopamine in the basal ganglia of the brain.

Once the diagnosis of Parkinson's disease is made, there is considerable variability in the course of the disease from one person to the next. However, there are some consistent themes. Symptoms begin in one limb only, most commonly an arm. This is referred to as "unilateral onset." At first, individuals respond well to treatment with dopamine agonists and/or dopamine replacement. On a practical level, this means that, when people are taking their medication, there is no visible rest tremor or slowness in their movement. To the untrained observer, there is no evidence of any sort of illness. During this period, which typically spans the first seven to eight years after diagnosis, the symptoms slowly spread to other parts of the body. For example, a rest tremor that was only present in the right arm will appear in the right leg. Gradually, the left arm and/or left leg will become affected as well. Despite the spread of symptoms, they continue to be well controlled with medication. However, after seven or eight years, complications typically develop. In broad terms, these complications can be divided into those affecting mobility, termed motor complications, and those affecting mood, sleep, and cognition, termed nonmotor complications. We will discuss each of these complications and potential treatments below. In Chapter 9, we will review some fictional case studies and discuss the ways in which the various symptoms of Parkinson's disease can be relieved, in practical terms.

MOTOR COMPLICATIONS

Wearing Off

Over time, the duration of relief that a person gets from anti-Parkinson medications becomes shorter and shorter. This is termed "wearing off" and is one of the most common motor complications of Parkinson's disease. In the early stage of Parkinson's disease, which can last for many years, an individual usually takes medication three to four times a day. Occasionally, one may forget to take a dose without experiencing a significant worsening of symptoms. Often, those in the early stages of Parkinson's disease do not notice a significant worsening of symptoms unless they skip an entire day of medication. As the disease progresses, however, the same person who used to forget to take an occasional dose begins to take the medication precisely at the prescribed times. This usually occurs because he or she can sense that the stiffness or tremor is returning in the hour before the next dose is due. Some people do not notice the return of a tremor but do feel as if their whole body "slows down" in the hour before the next dose of medication is due.

In some people, the wearing-off effect can be even more pronounced, especially in people who do not exhibit any visible signs of Parkinson's disease when their medication is working. In such persons, they usually move about without difficulty for four or five hours after taking a dose of medication. Then, they suddenly become stiff, slow, and have difficulty walking. In an "off" state, it is also common for people to feel anxious and be slower in processing information and responding to questions. It is not that they do not understand what is being asked or what is going on around them, it is just that the brain is working slowly, like the body.

Let us discuss Louis, for example. Louis was diagnosed with Parkinson's disease four years ago. He is sixty-two years old and works as a tenth grade science teacher. His family knows that he has Parkinson's disease. At work, neither his fellow teachers nor his students have any idea that he has a chronic illness. This is because he carefully times his medications so that he gets optimal control of his symptoms while he is teaching. Louis takes medication when he first wakes up, so that he can shower and get dressed easily. Then, when he gets to school, he takes a dose of medication at 7:30 A.M. Classes begin at 8:15 A.M., and Louis teaches four classes in a row until 11:25 A.M., when he breaks for lunch. After the students leave his classroom, he pulls out a glass of water and his next dose of pills. He takes them, eats lunch, and teaches two more classes before the end of the day at 2:15 P.M. Louis takes one more dose of medication before he drives home. Louis is very careful about taking the medication on time, because of an experience he had in the previous school year.

In May, just before classes let out for the summer, Louis had dismissed his class and reached for his 11:30 A.M. dose of medication, to discover that he had forgotten to bring it to the classroom! He had been able to write on the chalkboard and walk around the room during his class, but by 11:25 A.M., when the bell rang, he could feel that his hands were stiffening. By 11:30 A.M., he could feel his legs stiffening and he began to feel "lousy" in general. He knew that he had the medication in his bag in the teacher's room. However, the teacher's room was fifty feet down the hall. He tried to stand up from his chair, but his feet "froze" and he was unable to move at all. He quickly sat back down and realized that his hands were beginning to shake. He pretended to be busy, shuffling papers on his desk so that the one student who was still in the room would not notice anything. He then told that student that he was feeling ill and asked her to get his bag from the teacher's room. She brought him the bag and then left the room. Although his hands were shaking, Louis was able to reach for his pill bottle without difficulty. He then took his medication and waited thirty minutes. He could feel the medication "kick in," because the shaking in his hands stopped and the general "lousy" feeling he had disappeared. He was then able to get up and walk down the hall, perfectly normally, to eat lunch.

The reason(s) behind the development of the wearing-off effect are not understood. It may be that, as the disease progresses, patients stop responding as well to the medication. It is thought that, with disease progression, more and more dopamine-producing neurons die. When the medication that serves to supplement the brain's dopamine levels declines, there is little naturally produced dopamine available. As a result, the patient then experiences a rapid decline in dopamine levels, resulting in a limited ability to move. Most likely, the changes in response to dopamine treatment that occur with time are the result of a complex interaction between the imperfect addition of dopamine in the form of oral medication and the ongoing loss of dopamine-producing nerve cells in the brain.

The wearing-off effect can be minimized. One approach is to use a longer acting form of carbidopa/levodopa, known as Sinemet CR. The CR stands for controlled release. The difference between a tablet of regular carbidopa/levodopa and a CR tablet is that the regular tablet is fully absorbed within one hour of it being taken, whereas the CR tablet takes longer, approximately two hours, to be fully absorbed. As a result, the peak level of dopamine occurs at a later time and lasts for a longer period when one takes the CR tablet than when one takes the regular tablet.

Another approach is to add a second drug, entacapone (Comtan), which prolongs the life of dopamine in the brain. For those who find it difficult to take both a Sinemet tablet and a Comtan tablet at the same time, there is a single tablet that contains all three medications (carbidopa, levodopa, and entacapone). This tablet is known as Stalevo. The advantage to using Stalevo is that one need only take one pill, instead of two. The disadvantage is that Stalevo is only available in three fixed doses, making it more difficult to tailor the precise amount of dopamine to the needs of each patient. Yet another choice is to continue to take only carbidopa/levodopa and increase the frequency of the doses. For example, a person might take carbidopa/levodopa every three to four hours rather than every six to eight hours.

Many people who experience wearing off learn to schedule their activities so that they are at home, or seated comfortably at work, when the medication is due to wear off. They also get into the habit of keeping an extra set of pills near the chair where they typically sit or in the drawer of a desk at work, along with a bottle of water. By keeping some pills nearby, they will not have to struggle to walk to the cabinet where the medication is kept as the medication is wearing off. Once the next dose of medication kicks in and someone is "on," movements are quite smooth and easy to initiate. It is not unusual for people to look and move essentially normally when they are "on," which is when the dose of dopamine is at its peak in the body.

Dystonia

Dystonia is the uncontrolled contraction of agonist and antagonist muscles, resulting in an abnormal posture in the affected body region. Dystonia can involve any part of the body, such as a foot, the trunk, or neck. Dystonic contractions and their resulting abnormal postures can be painful and protracted. In those with Parkinson's disease, dystonia tends to occur when levels of dopamine rise or fall. The most common form of dystonia consists of end-of-dose foot cramps. Typically, in the hour before the next dose of carbidopa/levodopa is due to be taken, the toes curl under and the midportion of the foot becomes tight and stiff. Not only is this painful, but it makes walking difficult as well. In a sense, one can think of end-of-dose dystonia as a particularly severe form of the wearing-off effect. When dopamine levels are at their lowest, the muscles become so tight that cramps develop. End-of-dose dystonia can be easily remedied. One can minimize the risk of developing end-of-dose dystonia by either taking more tablets of carbidopa/levodopa, taken at shorter intervals during the day, or using a longer-acting form of carbidopa/levodopa.

A more difficult type of dystonia is that which occurs when dopamine levels are at their peak. The way in which high levels of dopamine result in dystonia is not understood. However, this form of dystonia typically occurs late in the course of Parkinson's disease, several years after end-of-dose dystonia is experienced. It is likely that peak-dose dystonia occurs as the result of a complex interplay between declining endogenous dopamine production, changes in dopamine receptors that occur as the disease progresses, and the imperfect supplementation of dopamine via medication. Peak-dose dystonia is difficult to treat. To treat peak-dose dystonia, one must reduce the total amount of dopamine taken during a day. The problem with this treatment is that it will result in a worsening of the other symptoms of Parkinson's disease: bradykinesia, rigidity, and rest tremor. Unfortunately, there is no treatment that is specific for peak-dose dystonia.

Dyskinesias

Dyskinesias are rapid, uncontrolled movements that involve the arms, legs, trunk, or head. The movements usually involve the entire limb or trunk and consist of writhing or persistent snake-like movements. Dyskinesias usually develop seven to eight years after Parkinson's disease is diagnosed. Dyskinesias usually occur when levels of dopamine are at their peak. Unlike dystonia, which can be quite painful, people often find dyskinesias more emotionally upsetting than physically uncomfortable. Given the choice between experiencing uncontrolled movements versus not being able to move at all, many people with Parkinson's disease prefer to err on the side of dyskinesias. Frequently, those watching someone who is dyskinetic feel uncomfortable and have an urge to do something to stop the uncontrolled movements. It is important to keep in mind that a medication regimen is adjusted for the benefit of the individual with Parkinson's disease, not for those around them. However, depending on their severity, dyskinesias can also be disabling, exhausting, and upsetting to the person with Parkinson's disease.

The way in which dyskinesias develop is poorly understood. What is clear, however, is that the two main factors that contribute to the development of dyskinesias are the level of dopamine in the brain at a given time and the severity of the Parkinson's disease itself. It seems as if a combination of these two factors leads to changes in the brain that result in dyskinesias. As in the case of peak-dose dystonia, it is a combination of disease severity and imperfect dopamine supplementation, in the form of oral medication, that is thought to contribute to the development of dyskinesias. Based on this limited understanding of how dyskinesias develop, physicians have developed several strategies in an attempt to delay their onset.

One strategy is to delay the onset of dopamine supplementation. Once dopamine supplementation is clearly required to help control the symptoms of Parkinson's disease, this approach recommends using as small a daily dose as possible. The problem with this strategy is that delaying the use of or using only small amounts of dopamine may not adequately control the symptoms of Parkinson's disease. This may result in a persistent rest tremor or marked walking difficulties that may lead to a fall and significant injury.

Yet another strategy is to smooth out the levodopa dose throughout the day, minimizing the number of peaks and valleys in brain dopamine concentration. The rationale behind this strategy is that dyskinesias develop because of adaptations the brain makes to rapid shifts in the levels of available dopamine. Practically speaking, this means taking pills more frequently throughout the day. Although this can be inconvenient, it does help to maximize mobility throughout the day. However, there is not any data to support the hypothesis that smoothing out the levodopa dose on a daily basis will minimize dyskinesias seven to eight years after Parkinson's disease is diagnosed.

A third strategy for managing dyskinesias is to add the drug amantadine (Symmetrel) to the daily drug regimen. No one understands the way in which amantadine works in the brain of someone with Parkinson's disease. However, it is clear that amantadine does help to reduce the severity of dyskinesias. The most prominent side effect of amantadine that limits the amount that can be used is some confusion or "dulling" of the thought processes.

Despite concerns over the role that long-term levodopa use may have in the development of dyskinesias, it is important to remember that our understanding of how dyskinesias develop is imperfect. A person with Parkinson's disease should not delay taking levodopa if they find that their Parkinson's symptoms make it difficult to participate in regular activities.

Skipped-Dose Phenomena

Some people may occasionally find that a particular dose of medication is not effective at all. This is known as the "skipped-dose phenomenon" and typically occurs on a random basis. One method for minimizing the risk of experiencing a skipped dose is to reduce the amount of protein that is eaten in the hour before a dose of levodopa is taken. In the intestines, the same pump mechanism that is used to absorb protein also absorbs levodopa. If someone eats a high-protein meal within forty-five minutes of having taken a dose of levodopa, the amount of levodopa that gets absorbed into the body may be less than if they had eaten a low-protein meal. A common strategy that is used to maximize the amount of levodopa that is absorbed is to limit the amount of protein eaten at breakfast and lunch. In this manner, the absorption of and response to levodopa is maximized during the day. Dinner can then contain a relatively high amount of protein. However, the amount of levodopa that is absorbed in the evenings may be reduced on such a diet. This dietary plan is feasible only if one is most active during the day and at home and minimally active at night. In addition, weight loss and malnutrition are significant risks of the low-protein diet. No diet should be initiated without first consulting one's physician.

NONMOTOR COMPLICATIONS

The nonmotor complications of Parkinson's disease encompass all the symptoms that are not directly related to motor tone or ease of movement. This category of symptoms includes sleep abnormalities, cognitive abnormalities, and changes in behavior or personality. This is an area that is receiving increased attention from physicians, scientists, and pharmaceutical companies. At academic medical centers, research is being conducted to identify and understand the types of nonmotor symptoms that are seen in those with Parkinson's disease. In pharmaceutical companies, work is being conducted to identify drugs that can help to relieve these nonmotor symptoms. Thus, our knowledge about these problems and potential treatments that are specific for each of them will likely expand in the coming years.

Sleep

To understand the abnormalities in sleep that are found in Parkinson's disease, it helps to first understand what is known about a healthy sleep pattern. Sleep is a complex, active event involving the brain. Sleep is subdivided into two general states: nonrapid eye movement sleep (NREM) and rapid eye movement sleep (REM). REM is also known as stage 5 sleep.

NREM sleep accounts for about three-fourths of our sleep cycle and consists of four stages. Stage 1 is the lightest stage of sleep. Stage 1 sleep encompasses the transition from wakefulness to deeper sleep. Stage 1 sleep lasts for about ten minutes. While in stage 1 sleep, a person can be easily woken. Stage 2 is known as intermediate sleep. During stage 2 sleep, eye movement stops. Stage 2 sleep accounts for 40 to 50 percent of total sleep time in young adults. Sleep stages 3 and 4 are known as deep sleep and typically account for 20 percent of total sleep time in young adults. As people get older, the amount of time spent in sleep stages 3 and 4 decreases. The function of NREM sleep is unknown.

REM sleep is the period during which there is dreaming and associated rapid bursts of eye movement. Although the true function of REM sleep is uncertain, rats that are totally deprived of REM sleep for several weeks will die. Clearly, REM sleep is an essential life-sustaining function.

The stages of sleep occur in cycles lasting 90–120 minutes each. Thus, four to five complete cycles occur during a typical night of sleep. During the first 90 minutes of sleep, an individual passes from wakefulness into stage 1 sleep and then to stages 2–4. The individual then returns first to stage 3 sleep and then to stage 2 sleep. After this, REM sleep is seen for the first time. As the night progresses, stage 2 sleep and REM sleep alternate until it is time to wake up.

In people with sleep disorders, the normal sleep cycle is disrupted and the number of changes from one stage of sleep to another increases. Keep in mind that people with Parkinson's disease tend to be older (that is, over sixty years of age). Aging itself affects the sleep cycle. As we age, the amount of time that we spend in the deep sleep of stages 3 and 4 declines, whereas stage 1 sleep (light sleep) increases. Thus, people with Parkinson's disease experience sleep difficulties as a result of both their age and their disease. This combination can result in a significant disruption of the normal sleep cycle, leaving a person feeling tired all of the time.

There is growing evidence that dopamine plays a complex role in the physiology of the sleep-wake cycle. Thus, in Parkinson's disease, it is not surprising that, as dopamine-producing brain cells die, the sleep-wake cycle is disrupted. Studies done in people with Parkinson's disease have shown abnormalities in stages 3 and 4 and REM sleep.

In normal REM sleep, our muscles are essentially paralyzed. This means that the dreams that occur during REM sleep are not acted out. People with Parkinson's disease, however, may develop a REM disorder. This means that muscle activity is not inhibited during dreams and excessive motor activity occurs. During truly vivid dreams, the motor activity can be so prominent that a person injures himself or herself and even a bedmate. This is in stark contrast to the symptoms of Parkinson's disease seen when someone is awake, when motor activity is difficult to initiate.

A variety of anti-Parkinson drugs can contribute to sleep disruptions. Selegiline (Deprenyl) and amantadine (Symmetrel) are two that can increase nighttime wakefulness. Other medications, such as ropinirole (Requip) and pramipexole (Mirapex), have been implicated in excessive daytime sleepiness. Thus, both the underlying Parkinson's disease and the medications used to alleviate its symptoms may result in sleep abnormalities.

The question of daytime sleepiness in Parkinson's disease is controversial and complicated to analyze. There have been reports that some of the anti-Parkinson medications are the cause of "sleep attacks" that have resulted in car accidents in otherwise seemingly competent patients. The dopamine agonists ropinirole (Requip) and pramipexole (Mirapex) have been implicated as causing these "sleep attacks." However, people with Parkinson's disease have many reasons to be sleepy during the day. The disruptions in the normal sleep cycle, which are the result of both their age and the underlying Parkinson's disease, contribute to a sensation of persistent fatigue and a tendency to nap during the day. Depression, which is seen in many with Parkinson's disease, also disrupts the normal sleep cycle and can also contribute to daytime sleepiness. In summary, it is clear that Parkinson's disease results in fragmented sleep patterns. However, it is not yet clear precisely how Parkinson's disease affects sleep and how best to treat these sleep abnormalities that are caused by Parkinson's disease. It is also not clear how some of the medications used to treat Parkinson's disease affect the sleep cycle. Sleep research, and in particular the effect of Parkinson's disease on the sleep cycle, is an area of active research.

Cognition

The term cognition encompasses all the mental processes that a person uses in gathering and using information. Cognitive function can be broken down into several different components, including visuospatial skill, executive function, attention, the ability to store and retrieve information, and language processing. In Parkinson's disease, some of these elements of cognition are affected whereas others are not. Many psychological tests are available to measure the degree of decline in cognitive ability and which components of cognition are affected. When a doctor asks a patient to undergo detailed cognitive testing, the goal is to use the results to determine the type of cognitive deficits and to help in making a clinical diagnosis. For example, the pattern of cognitive changes in Parkinson's disease is very different from that seen in Alzheimer's disease. People with Alzheimer's disease have difficulty with language processing and retrieving information. These are cognitive domains that remain intact in those with Parkinson's disease. This difference in cognitive dysfunction likely reflects the difference in the areas of the brain that are affected in these two distinct diseases.

Dementia is not a specific disease. Dementia is a term used to describe a group of symptoms in which there is a decline in brain function that affects a person's ability to think clearly and perform normal activities, such as driving, cooking, and getting dressed. Many different medical disorders can cause dementia. The behavioral characteristics and changes in cognitive function that are seen vary, depending on the particular type of dementia that a person has.

In Parkinson's disease, research indicates that some cognitive domains are more likely to be affected than others. The onset of the cognitive symptoms is usually slow. The cognitive domains that are most often affected include attention, memory and learning, executive functions, and visuospatial functions. Verbal function and the ability to reason seem to be spared, although information processing may be slower. Slowed information processing is referred to as bradyphrenia, with "brady-" meaning slow (as in bradykinesia, or slow movement) and "-phrenia" referring to the head.

Attention

This refers to the ability to focus and concentrate on a specific stimulus, sensation, idea, or thought. It applies to the ability to focus and concentrate on things that are presented visually or verbally. Attention and concentration are essential to one's ability to remember and plan.

Memory

Memory is the store of knowledge that we acquire through experience. Memory can be divided into free recall and cued recall. Free recall is the ability to retrieve information independently. For example, the ability to retrieve dates and events for an essay that is part of a history exam requires the use of free recall. Cued recall is the ability to retrieve information when it is presented in a helpful context. For example, the ability to correctly identify the name of one's fifth grade teacher, when given a list of possible names, requires the use of cued recall.

Executive Functions

These are the mental processes involved in goal-directed behavior. Goal-directed behavior can be divided into two subsets, those that are internally guided and those that are externally guided. People with Parkinson's disease generally have problems with internally guided behavior but the externally guided behavior is normal.

For example, Mary is seventy-five years old and was diagnosed with Parkinson's disease seven years ago. She is babysitting her grandson, Jason, who is ten years old. It is Saturday night, and Jason would like to have pizza for dinner. Jason tells his grandmother about a nearby pizzeria, Antonio's. Jason thinks that Antonio's makes great pepperoni pizza. He also knows that they will deliver the pizza to their home. Armed with this information, Mary is able to find the phone number for Antonio's, call them, and order a pizza to be delivered. This is an example of externally guided behavior. It is Jason who decided what to eat and how to get it. With those choices made, Mary had no difficulty in ordering the pizza.

Let us now consider a different scenario. Mary is back in her own home, where she lives alone. It is six o'clock on a Saturday evening, and Mary has nothing to do. She notices that her neighbors are barbecuing and realizes that it is time for dinner. Mary enters her kitchen and looks in the refrigerator, but she can't decide whether to cook the chicken legs or the pork chop that she finds. So, she pours herself a glass of lemonade and starts to watch television. The next thing she knows, it is eight o'clock and she is feeling hungry but cannot decide what to eat. This is an example of a lack of internally guided behavior. Left on her own, Mary cannot decide when to eat or what to eat.

In addition to difficulties with internally guided behavior, other executive functions are affected in Parkinson's disease as well. The ability to maintain an attention set and adapt to a changing environment are also affected. An attention set refers to the ability to focus on a specific project or stimulus until it is complete or fully processed. For example, a healthy sixteen year old will be able to clean their bedroom and do their own laundry in two hours, all while listening to their favorite music on an iPod. In contrast, a woman who is sixty-two years old and has Parkinson's disease will have to turn off any music, as well as the television, to clean the bedroom without getting distracted.

Set shifting refers to the ability to change one's thought processes based on changes in the environment. For example, when the cost of gas is low, people tend to buy larger cars, such as sports utility vehicles. When the cost of gas is high, people tend to buy smaller compact cars. This is an example of set shifting. Someone with Parkinson's disease has difficulty changing their behavior based on changes in the environment. Thus, someone with Parkinson's disease who bought a large car when gas prices were low would go out and buy another such vehicle, even if the price of gas has tripled.

Visuospatial Functions

People with Parkinson's disease have visuospatial deficits that are distinct from their motor abnormalities. Examples of visuospatial skills in everyday life include the ability to draw a map showing how to get from one's house to the shopping mall, set the table for dinner, and tie shoelaces. People with Parkinson's disease may have trouble with one or all of these tasks.

Cognitive functions are measured by using paper and pencil tests or by having a person take the tests on a computer. Testing is usually performed by a specially trained psychologist and takes several hours. The patient is asked to answer some questions verbally, whereas other segments of the test require putting puzzles together or arranging blocks to match a drawing. Reading and writing tasks may also be part of the testing.

In one study of people who had mild Parkinson's disease, researchers found that 36 percent showed some form of cognitive impairment (Athey, Porter, and Walker 2005, 268). Specifically, these patients had difficulty with visual processing and executive functioning. In another study, conducted in people whose Parkinson's disease was more advanced, testing showed that 23 percent of the subjects had marked difficulty with memory and abstract thinking (Foltynie et al. 2004, 550). Unfortunately, these two studies used different tests of cognitive ability. Thus, we cannot directly compare the results of the study done on people whose Parkinson's disease was relatively mild to the results of the study done on people whose Parkinson's disease was more advanced.

To fully understand the cognitive changes that are associated with Parkinson's disease, additional research is needed. Ideally, a large group of patients with Parkinson's disease should be followed from the time of diagnosis until their death, with systematic cognitive testing performed once every two to three years. Armed with such data regarding the severity of cognitive dysfunction and the specific thought processes that are affected, scientists and physicians can then consider developing treatments that are specific to the cognitive deficits found in Parkinson's disease.

In summary, the most commonly identified cognitive problems in people with Parkinson's disease are decreases in attention, executive function, and visuospatial function. Language, the ability to recognize people and things, and reasoning tend to be less affected or unaffected by Parkinson's disease.

Treatment of Cognitive Dysfunction Associated with Parkinson's Disease

Managing the symptoms of cognitive dysfunction in Parkinson's patients can be quite complicated. The doctor may want to evaluate the current medications that are being used. This is because some of the medications used to treat Parkinson's disease, such as amantadine (Symmetrel), can cause confusion. Giving medication that may result in confusion as a side effect, to someone who has cognitive problems as a result of their disease, can significantly worsen their abilities. Typically, however, it is impractical to discontinue the anti-Parkinson medications, because this will worsen one's mobility. The doctor will probably withdraw nonessential medications from the patient's regimen slowly and in a particular order, to look for signs of improvement in cognitive function. Unfortunately, there is no medication that is specific for the treatment of the cognitive abnormalities found in Parkinson's disease.

Mood

Many people with Parkinson's disease experience depression. About half of the people with Parkinson's disease have a form of depression called dysthymia. It is a common and mild form of depression that, if left untreated, may become chronic and long lasting. A person with dysthymia goes through the day functioning at a less than an optimal level. The symptoms of dysthymia vary from person to person but may include any combination of the following symptoms: lowered self-esteem, feelings of guilt, persistent self-critical thoughts, difficulty concentrating or making decisions, feelings of hopelessness, tearful episodes, a change in eating or sleeping habits, reckless behavior, and a low energy level.

Major depression is common in people with Parkinson's disease. The symptoms of major depression are similar to dysthymia but more pronounced, in that they significantly interfere with a person's ability to eat, enjoy life, concentrate on a task, and sleep.

Researchers think that one of the primary causes of depression is that there is a relatively low level of serotonin in the brain. Serotonin is a neurotransmitter that is released from neurons to stimulate other neurons. Normally, serotonin is released from one neuron and enters the synapse. The synapse is the

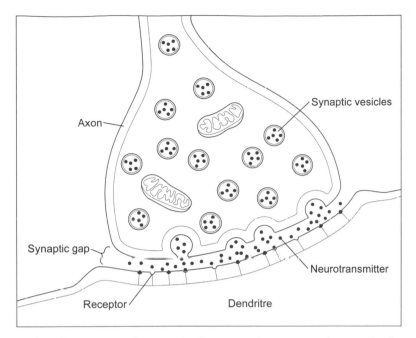

Figure 5.1. A synapse is the specialized junction between two brain cells through which the cells signal to one another. Neurotransmitters are stored, in vesicles, and are released into the synaptic gap when the brain cell is stimulated. The transmitters travel across the synaptic gap and bind to specific receptors in the neighboring cell, resulting in changes within that cell. *Illustrated by Jeff Dixon.*

space between adjacent neurons, in which they communicate with each other (see Figure 5.1). In the case of a neuron that produces serotonin, the neuron communicates with its neighbor by releasing serotonin into the synapse. The serotonin diffuses across the synapse and binds to its receptors on the neighboring cell. A series of changes occur within the second neuron, in response to the fact that serotonin has bound to its receptors on the cell surface. This second cell then goes on to send signals to other cells. In the meantime, the serotonin that had bound to its receptor on the neighboring cell gets released back into the synapse. The free serotonin now suffers one of two fates. Some of the serotonin is degraded and the rest returns to the cell that released it, in which it is taken up and repackaged. The serotonin will then be stored within the cell until it is released again, to send another message to another cell. This is the way in which brain cells communicate with one another and is referred to as neurotransmission.

In people with depression, scientists hypothesize that serotonin is not released properly or is present in low levels. It was this hypothesis that led to the development of the antidepressant drugs known as the SSRIs. These medications prevent the return, or reuptake, of serotonin into the cell from which it was released. By allowing serotonin to remain in the synapse for a longer period, it will bind to more receptors and send out a "stronger" signal than if it had been repackaged quickly. The result is that other brain cells will think that there is more serotonin being released, which results in an improved mood.

In addition to its effects on mood, serotonin also plays a role in regulating the release of dopamine. Studies have shown that people with Parkinson's disease have a lowered level of serotonin in their brain. There is evidence that this decrease in serotonin might be caused by the low levels of dopamine in those with Parkinson's disease. This suggests a feedback mechanism between the brain cells that produce serotonin and the ones that produce dopamine. Based on the evidence available, scientists hypothesize that the low levels of dopamine that are seen in the brain of someone with Parkinson's disease send a message to the serotonin-producing cells, telling them to produce less serotonin. With less serotonin, the chance of developing depression increases.

Does this mean that someone with depression is at risk of developing Parkinson's disease? The short answer is no. There is no evidence that depression is a risk factor for Parkinson's disease. However, it is known that depression is more common in people with Parkinson's disease. The hypothesis discussed here, regarding the interplay between dopamine and serotonin levels, provides a framework in which to think about the interactions between various neurotransmitters, and the symptoms that result, in those with Parkinson's disease.

In 2002, research supporting the link between depression and Parkinson's disease was published in the scientific journal *Neurology*. These data were also presented at the annual meeting of the American Academy of Neurology. The American Academy of Neurology is a medical specialty society dedicated to advancing the field of neurology. It supports both basic science and clinical research in the field of neurology. It also provides continuing medication education for practicing neurologists. The journal *Neurology* is published by the American Academy of Neurology. All papers submitted to the journal are carefully reviewed, by unbiased experts in the field, before their acceptance for publication. The process whereby scientific data is reviewed before publication is known as "peer review." Thus, those reports that are published in journals that use peer review have already been critically assessed for study design, quality of the results, and validity of the conclusions that are made. In general, conclusions that are based on data that are published in a journal that uses the peer review process is more likely to be accurate than conclusions presented in other forums that do not use peer review.

In the report regarding depression and Parkinson's disease, researchers began with a health directory containing medical information about all the patients seen by general practitioners in fifty-three different medical practices in The Netherlands (Schuurman et al. 2002, 1501). They identified the patients who had symptoms of depression. The health directory contained records of nearly 69,000 people. Of this group, 1,358 fit the strict criteria for depression. They could not be psychotic and must have experienced at least three of the following six feelings: (1) sadness or melancholy more than can be explained by psychosocial stress, (2) suicidal thoughts or attempts, (3) indecisiveness, decreased interest in usual activities, or diminished ability to think, (4) feelings of worthlessness, self-reproach, or inappropriate or excessive guilt, (5) early morning awakening, excessive sleeping, or early morning fatigue, and (6) anxiety, extreme irritability, or agitation.

In the depressed group of subjects, nineteen people developed Parkinson's disease. In the nondepressed group of subjects, 259 people developed Parkinson's disease. Converting to percentages, 1.4 percent of people in the depressed group developed Parkinson's disease compared with 0.4 percent in the nondepressed group. This might not sound like much of a difference, but, in epidemiological terms, the results are significantly different. This indicates that there is a significant connection between depression and Parkinson's disease.

There are unique characteristics to the depression found in those with Parkinson's disease. Specifically, depressed patients with Parkinson's disease experience higher rates of anxiety, are more often sad without feeling guilt or self-blame, and have lower rates of suicide despite higher rates of suicidal thoughts.

Depression, whether it is diagnosed in those with Parkinson's disease or not, is not only common but it is also treatable. Thanks to the availability of a wide range of effective antidepressant medications, no one needs to suffer through its uncomfortable symptoms. There are several different classes of antidepressant medications. Thus, if a person cannot tolerate the side effects of one type of antidepressant, there are other several other options available. It is important to understand that depression has biochemical origins. The reason that medications are effective in treating depression is that they target the problem in the cells of the brain that produce the chemicals that help control our mood. Taking a medication for depression is similar to taking a medication for pneumonia or asthma. All of these medications act on the underlying biologic or biochemical cause of the disorder being treated.

Mental health professionals are the best source for information about and the treatment of depression. There are many different specialists working in the field of mental health, including medical doctors, psychologists, and social workers. A psychiatrist has an M.D. and received his or her training in a medical school and hospital. A psychologist holds a master's degree or a Ph.D. from a university. In some states, one must have a Ph.D. degree to call oneself a psychologist, whereas in other states someone with a master's degree in psychology can advertise as a psychologist. A social worker typically holds a bachelor's or master's degree from a school of social work. Essentially, two different types of treatment are used for depression: psychotherapy and antidepressant medication. Most patients do best using both types of treatment at the same time.

Psychotherapy

Psychotherapies encompass several different types of talk therapies in which patients describe and discuss troubling events in their lives. A patient works with a therapist to understand or change the way he or she reacts to events. Three common styles of psychotherapy are cognitive/behavioral therapy, interpersonal therapy, and psychodynamic therapy. The use of one type of talk therapy does not preclude the use of others. Many therapists mingle elements of all three styles of psychotherapy depending on the needs of a particular patient. Most talk therapies consist of weekly sessions held for about ten to twenty weeks. Each therapy session is usually forty-five to fifty minutes in length.

Cognitive/behavioral therapy helps people understand how their feelings and behavior can be influenced by the way they think. Say, for example, that you must give an oral presentation, in front of your political science class, about the end of the cold war. On the day of the presentation, your stomach is rumbling and you feel a little nauseous. Most people would assume that these symptoms are the result of feeling nervous and afraid. Why not assume that they are attributable to being excited and eager instead? Notice how using more upbeat adjectives give the stomach sensation a positive and more pleasant twist. Cognitive/behavioral therapy helps patients identify patterns of thought and behavior that can contribute to depression. The goal is to eliminate those thought and behavior patterns, thus lessening the severity of the depression.

Interpersonal therapy explores a person's relationships with relatives; friends, colleagues, and even strangers to find patterns that might be triggering or contributing to the depression. This therapeutic approach assumes that there is a connection between mood and relationships and that aspects of one's relationships are contributing to depression. Thus, mood will improve once the maladaptive relationship pattern is identified and changed.

Psychodynamic therapy evolved from the Freudian style of psychoanalytic therapy. Sigmund Freud was an Austrian doctor who founded the field of psychoanalysis. Psychoanalysis is a treatment in which the doctor, who is also referred to as an analyst, listens to the patient describe his or her thoughts and behaviors. The doctor then explains, to the patient, the unconscious basis for their behavior and mood problems.

Psychodynamic therapy as practiced today is usually shorter term than what Freud used and focuses on a specific problem such as depression rather than on the whole personality. The therapist tries to help the patient identify the underlying causes of his or her problem. This approach explores a person's past to learn what events led up to the current emotional state. It assumes that emotions drive actions and that understanding the underlying emotion will allow a person to make changes and eliminate the cause of the depression.

Is talk therapy of any type really effective? It is most effective when the psychotherapist and patient have a good working relationship and the patient understands that there is effort involved in feeling better. Here are some of the ways psychotherapy is effective for overcoming depression: it pinpoints life problems that contribute to depression; it explores negative or distorted patterns of thought and behavior that contribute to feelings of despair and helplessness; it helps a person understand which aspects of the problems can be solved or improved; it identifies realistic goals for improving emotional well-being; and it helps people regain a sense of control and pleasure in life.

Antidepressant Medications

Medications can be very effective in managing depression, particularly when the depression is moderate, severe, or chronic. Treatment that uses a combination of talk therapy and antidepressant drugs is common and has been shown to be more effective than using either treatment modality alone. Antidepressant medications take several weeks, at least, to reach their maximum effectiveness. Typically, the dose of antidepressant medication is adjusted over several months as an individual undergoes psychotherapy. People who are diagnosed with dysthymia, the persistent sensation of feeling low and out of sorts, are excellent candidates for treatment with antidepressant medications. In addition, those whose symptoms continue for several weeks or who are not responding to talk therapy are excellent candidates for antidepressant medication. When the question of depression arises in someone with Parkinson's disease, it is important to discuss it with the neurologist who is taking care of the patient.

The most commonly prescribed antidepressants for people with Parkinson's disease are the SSRIs. This class of medications includes drugs such as fluoxetine (Prozac), sertraline (Zoloft), citalopram (Celexa), paroxetine (Paxil), and fluvoxamine (Luvox). The older antidepressants such as amitriptyline (Elavil) or nortriptyline (Pamelor), which are in a category known as the tricyclic antidepressants (TCAs), are also an option and are sometimes prescribed instead of the SSRIs. In addition, there are several relatively new antidepressant medications that are not classified as either SSRIs or tricyclics. Buproprion (Wellbutrin), for example, is an effective antidepressant. Another alternative for the treatment of depression is mirtazapine (Remeron).

Millions of people worldwide use medication for the treatment of depression, and the effect has been quite remarkable. Most report that they feel better and become more productive. In fact, studies indicate that 35–45 percent of people who take an SSRI experience complete resolution of their symptoms.

The SSRIs are not perfect, and side effects can limit their use. Not everyone experiences side effects, but for those who do, they may feel caught between two difficult choices: improving their mood but coping with unwanted side effects of the medication or remaining in a depressed state but without any additional, new physical problems. The short-term side effects of the SSRIs include dry mouth, jumpiness, headache, and stomach distress. These tend to be mild and resolve within a few weeks, once the body adapts to the medication. Longer-lasting side effects of the SSRIs include weight gain, loss of interest in sex, inability to achieve orgasm, insomnia, and memory lapses. It is important to remember that these side effects are reversible and disappear once the medication is no longer used. Not all the drugs have the same effect in every patient, so a doctor usually works closely with a patient to find the one that is most effective with the least number of side effects.

There can be a problem when certain SSRIs are given to some people with Parkinson's disease. Unlike the older types of antidepressant drugs that were sedating, some SSRIs can cause increased activity. That can be good news for people who are depressed and withdrawn but quite the opposite for someone who has a tendency to become agitated. Some people with Parkinson's disease also experience anxiety. In these patients, the choice of which SSRI to use must be made carefully. It is important to avoid those SSRIs that cause a general activation in their activity level, because this can result in worsening anxiety.

A second potential problem with the use of SSRIs in those with Parkinson's disease is a potential drug interaction. Some people with Parkinson's disease take selegiline (Deprenyl) to control their symptoms of Parkinson's. The manufacturers of SSRIs recommend against the combination of an SSRI and selegiline because of a potential for an adverse biochemical effect. This effect is referred to as the serotonin syndrome and may include irritability, hyperthermia, increased muscle tone, and altered consciousness.

Table 5.1.
Antidepressant Medications Commonly Used in Parkinson's Disease Patients

Trade name	Generic name	Drug class
Prozac	fluoxetine	SSRI
Paxil	paroxetine	SSRI
Zoloft	sertraline	SSRI
Luvox	fluvoxamine	SSRI
Celexa	citalopram	SSRI
Elavil	amitriptyline	TCA
Pamelor	nortriptyline	TCA
Tofranil	imipramine	TCA
Effexor	venlafaxine	Atypical antidepressant
Wellbutrin	bupropion	Atypical antidepressant
Remeron	mirtazapine	Atypical antidepressant

Despite these caveats, doctors do prescribe SSRIs to their patients with Parkinson's disease, and most are satisfied with the outcome. The decision of whether or not to treat depression and the choice of which antidepressant to use should be made in close consultation with one's neurologist and psychiatrist (see Table 5.1). As you can see, the potential for interactions amongst various drugs makes it critical to ensure that all medications, whether prescription or over the counter, are reviewed with all of the physicians involved in someone's care.

Other Psychiatric Aspects of Parkinson's Disease

The primary pathology in Parkinson's disease is the degeneration of dopamine-producing cells in the substantia nigra. Without adequate levels of dopamine, the brain's ability to control movement is limited. Dopamine is also important for other brain functions, particularly the processing of sensory information and behavior. As drug doses increase to ease worsening motor symptoms, the effect on behavior and mood can become especially evident. Some people may experience hallucinations, delusions, agitation, mania, or confusion.

A hallucination is a false perception that occurs without any true sensory stimulus. For example, a person hears a voice when no one is speaking or sees someone standing in front of them when no one is there. The number of people with Parkinson's disease who experience hallucinations is not certain but may range from 30 to 70 percent, depending on the severity of disease. Typically, hallucinations develop ten to twelve years after the disease is diagnosed.

In those with Parkinson's disease, visual hallucinations are the most common type of hallucination that is experienced. They typically occur at night and are nonthreatening. For example, a long-dead family member may appear at the bedside and engage in conversation.

Some people with Parkinson's disease experience auditory and tactile hallucinations as well. Auditory hallucinations are those in which a person hears sounds or distinct voices that are not actually present. Tactile hallucinations are those in which a person feels a sensation that cannot be attributed to real stimuli. Hallucinations are more common in those who are older, those taking relatively high doses of anti-Parkinson drugs, and those who have some cognitive impairment. Patients often understand that their hallucinations are a side effect of the medications that allow them to move more easily. The fact that the medications that cause the hallucinations are helpful in other ways and that the hallucinations are typically not frightening means that most people with Parkinson's disease are willing to live with them.

Delusions are fixed, false beliefs for which there is no basis in reality. Delusions in Parkinson's disease usually manifest as a fear of being injured, followed or watched, or deceived. The prevalence of delusions among those with Parkinson's disease is estimated to range from 3 to 17 percent.

Agitation is a common behavioral problem that can occur in those with Parkinson's disease. It refers to uncharacteristic stubbornness, worrying, and nervousness. Signs of agitation may include irritability, repetitive questioning, refusal to cooperate, and pacing or other persistent, nonpurposeful activity. To manage or calm down someone who is agitated, it can be helpful to simplify the task the person is working on or find an interesting distraction. If these methods are not effective, then treatment with a low dose of an antianxiety medication may be helpful.

The medications that are used to treat Parkinson's disease have also been associated with mania. The characteristics of mania include euphoria, a feeling of high self-esteem, increased activity, a diminished need for sleep, and hypersexuality. Hypersexuality is defined as the exhibition of unusual or excessive concern with or indulgence in sexual activity.

Hallucinations, delusions, agitation, or mania do not occur in everyone with Parkinson's disease. If these symptoms do develop, they can be minimized. One method is to lower the dose of the drugs used to treat the Parkinson's disease, especially the evening dose. The reason for this is that hallucinations and agitation typically worsen at night, as the sun goes down. However, this will undoubtedly cause a return of the motor symptoms of Parkinson's disease. Alternatively, adding a low dose of one of the newer antipsychotic drugs, referred to as "atypical" antipsychotics, can be quite effective in controlling the behavioral problems without significantly worsening the motor symptoms of Parkinson's disease. Thus, a low dose of an atypical antipsychotic medicine can control behavior without making someone with Parkinson's disease slower or more rigid. Because confusion and agitation in someone with Parkinson's disease can take a tremendous toll on the entire family, it is important to remember that these behaviors can be controlled with medication.

In Case of Emergency

Emergencies associated with Parkinson's disease are rare. Parkinson's disease is a chronic illness, so changes occur slowly, over months to years, rather than over hours to days. That being said, one's response to medication will diminish over time. Movements that used to be faster and smoother after taking medication may appear to be slower and the limbs may feel more stiff. When this happens, it is important to contact one's neurologist. Changes can be made to the medication regimen, slowly over the course of several weeks to months, to improve mobility.

When someone with Parkinson's disease develops any other illness, such as a cold or the flu, the Parkinson's symptoms will get worse. In this situation, it is important not to make changes in the medications used to treat Parkinson's disease but to wait until the acute illness resolves. Any worsening of the symptoms of Parkinson's disease that occurs in the setting of an infection or other acute illness is not a sign that the Parkinson's disease is getting worse. It simply means that the body is under stress from the acute illness and cannot compensate as well for the symptoms of Parkinson's disease. Several weeks after the acute illness resolves, the symptoms of Parkinson's disease will return to baseline.

Lifespan

A common concern is whether or not having Parkinson's disease will shorten someone's life. Because of the rapid pace at which better treatments have been developed, there is no clear answer to this question. In addition, there is significant variability in the symptoms of Parkinson's disease that are experienced by any given person. For people whose symptoms do not progress rapidly and who begin to experience the symptoms of Parkinson's disease at a relatively older age, Parkinson's disease is not likely to shorten lifespan.

6

Complementary and Alternative Therapies for Parkinson's Disease

Complementary and alternative therapies have many definitions. Most simply stated, they are treatments that have not been scientifically tested. This also means that knowledgeable experts, who do not have any personal or professional interest in the outcome, have not reviewed the results of any studies that were conducted. NIH, which is the agency of the federal government that is responsible for biomedical research, divides alternative therapy into two parts: complementary medicine and alternative medicine. Complementary and alternative medicine are defined by NIH as follows: "a group of diverse medical and healthcare systems, practices, and products ... for most there are key questions that are yet to be answered through well-designed scientific studies—questions such as whether they are safe and whether they work for the diseases or medical conditions for which they are used" (http://nccam.nih.gov).

Complementary medicine complements conventional Western-style medicine and is used in addition to usual medical care. An example of complementary medicine is regular participation in a yoga class. It is thought that, for someone with hypertension, the practice of yoga, in addition to the daily ingestion of medication, helps to relieve stress and keep one's blood pressure low. The practice of combining Western-style medicine with complementary therapies for which there is reasonable scientific proof of effectiveness is referred to as "integrative medicine." Alternative medicine, in contrast, is a substitute for traditional medicine. An example of alternative medicine is going on a special diet to fight breast cancer rather than undergoing surgery, chemotherapy, or radiation.

THE USE OF COMPLEMENTARY MEDICINE IN PARKINSON'S DISEASE

People with Parkinson's disease frequently use complementary therapy. A study of Parkinson's patients by doctors in Baltimore and Boston found that 40 percent had used some form of complementary therapy in conjunction with traditional treatment. Over 70 percent of this group used more than one form of complementary therapy. The most common therapies used were vitamins and herbs, massage, and acupuncture. There are many examples of complementary therapies. Several of the more commonly used therapies are described here. They are vitamin E, coenzyme Q_{10}, massage, St. John's wort, and Chinese exercise modalities.

Vitamins

There is no solid, scientific evidence to support the intake of any specific vitamin or vitamin combination for the treatment of Parkinson's disease. In fact, taking excess amounts of some vitamins may interfere with the effectiveness of some anti-Parkinson medications. For example, vitamin B_6 (pyridoxine) at doses that exceed 10 mg a day can accelerate the breakdown of levodopa in the body, making it less effective. There are several other vitamins that, when taken at relatively high doses, can result in significant side effects. However, taking one multivitamin a day will not have any harmful effect on Parkinson's disease and may benefit one's overall health. To ensure that vitamin supplements are not harmful, it is important to discuss the use of all prescription and nonprescription pills with one's physician.

Vitamin E

Vitamin E belongs to a class of vitamins called antioxidants. As discussed in Chapter 1, antioxidants bind and stabilize free radicals. Free radicals are highly reactive chemical species that arise naturally in the body and brain during normal metabolism. Free radicals are dangerous and damage proteins inside of cells by a process referred to as oxidation. Under certain conditions, free radicals may increase in number and damage cells. Thus, antioxidants are important compounds that help to inactivate free radicals, thereby minimizing damage to cells.

One hypothesis regarding the onset of Parkinson's disease is that the presence of high levels of free radicals leads to the death of dopamine neurons. Thus, increasing the levels of antioxidants in the brain may help prevent or slow the progression of Parkinson's disease.

To examine this theory, the National Institute of Neurological Disorders and Stroke, a division of NIH that focuses on neurological diseases, funded a large study looking at the effects of selegeline (also called deprenyl) and vitamin E (also called tocopherol) on early Parkinson's disease. This study was referred to as DATATOP (Deprenyl and Tocopherol Antioxidative Therapy for Parkinson's Disease). The study involved more than 50 investigators over a five-year period. The results did not provide any evidence that vitamin E helped in slowing the early progression of Parkinson's disease.

Despite the findings of the DATATOP study, some scientists still hypothesize that vitamin E, a different antioxidant or a combination of antioxidants might be beneficial for those with Parkinson's disease. However, the reader should not use this information to justify purchasing and ingesting large amounts of vitamin E on a daily basis.

Vitamin E can be harmful as well as helpful. Vitamin E can interfere with anticoagulant medicines. Anticoagulants are medications that minimize the risk that the blood in our vessels will clot. For people who have had clots in their legs or lungs, treatment with anticoagulants is absolutely necessary so that they do not lose a limb or die. Thus, for these people, taking too much vitamin E could be life threatening. There is also some confusion regarding vitamin E and heart disease. Recently, conflicting evidence has been reported concluding that vitamin E either increases or decreases one's risk of developing heart disease. The bottom line is that vitamin E supplements should be taken only after consultation with one's physician and in carefully regulated doses.

Coenzyme Q_{10}

Coenzyme Q_{10} is referred to by many different names, including CoQ_{10}, Q_{10}, vitamin Q_{10}, ubiquinone, and ubidecarenone. Coenzyme Q_{10} is made naturally by the body. Coenzyme Q_{10} is also an antioxidant. In addition to serving as an antioxidant, Coenzyme Q_{10} also helps cells produce the energy needed for their normal growth and maintenance.

Coenzyme Q_{10} is present in most places in the body, especially the heart, liver, kidneys, and pancreas. Scientists have found that people with Parkinson's disease have reduced levels of Q_{10} in specialized structures inside cells called mitochondria. Mitochondria are necessary for producing energy in cells. Without energy, cells cannot remain alive and healthy.

In a study of eighty people with Parkinson's disease, investigators at the University of California at San Diego found that patients taking a daily dose of 1200 mg of Q_{10} for a 16 month period scored significantly better on a Parkinson's disease rating scale at the end of the 16 month period than those who took either a lower dose of Q_{10} or a placebo. A placebo is a tablet that looks like the medication being tested but has no biological effects.

The rating scale that was used measured cognitive function and mood, activities of daily living, and motor skills. As we discussed previously, these are the areas that are affected by Parkinson's disease. Although this result is promising, the number of people in the study was relatively small. Thus, the results may be misleading. A larger group of patients are currently participating in a trial with Q_{10} to help determine whether the supplement is truly effective in treating Parkinson's disease.

Anyone who is considering using Q_{10} should talk with his or her physician. Q_{10} can interact with certain prescription medicines, which can reduce the effect of the supplement or the medication. For example, Q_{10} can change the body's response to insulin (which can cause serious side effects in diabetics) and certain anticoagulant medicines. Again, just as recommended with vitamin E, Q_{10} supplements should be taken only after consultation with one's physician and in carefully regulated doses.

Massage

Massage therapy is manual soft tissue manipulation, in which the goal is to improve the patient's health and sense of well-being. Does massage therapy benefit people with Parkinson's disease? Some people find that it helps relieve muscle stiffness and provides both physical and mental relaxation. Biologically, massage therapy claims to reduce heart rate, increase blood and lymph circulation in muscles, relax muscles, reduce soreness, improve range of motion, and increase endorphins. Endorphins are neurotransmitters that produce a sense of happiness or well-being when they are released. However, these claims have yet to be proven in rigorous, scientific trials.

The most common type of massage therapy is the Swedish massage. The therapist uses long strokes and kneading and friction techniques to stimulate surface muscles. The massage is combined with active and passive movement of the joints. Other types of massage therapy, such as rolfing or sports massage, use deep muscle massage techniques that can be somewhat painful. Shiatsu and acupressure massage therapies use finger pressure, which is thought to stimulate channels of energy flow throughout the body.

St. John's Wort

St. John's wort is a plant, also known as *Hypericum perforatum*. Many people use St. John's wort as an alternative therapy for treating their depression. That means that they will take St. John's wort rather than a prescription, antidepressant medication such as one of the SSRIs. As discussed in Chapter 4, the SSRIs are the most commonly prescribed antidepressant medications in the United States. Evidence from test tube experiments indicates that St. John's wort contains chemicals that act in a similar manner as the SSRIs. Does this mean that St. John's wort relieves depression? A European study published in 1996 in the *British Medical Journal* analyzed the outcome of twenty-three clinical trials of St. John's wort for the treatment of depression. Their results indicate that, for mild to moderate depression, St. John's wort works better than a placebo.

In major depression, however, there is conflicting evidence regarding the efficacy of St. John's wort. Several of these studies were not well designed or did not study the effects of St. John's wort in enough people. To date, there is no evidence to support the use of St. John's wort in the treatment of major depression and limited evidence to support its use in the treatment of mild to moderate depression. The efficacy of St. John's wort for the treatment of depression requires additional study. In the meantime, as discussed in Chapter 4, depression is best treated with the established therapies: prescription antidepressants and talk therapy.

The U.S. Food and Drug Administration (FDA) classifies St. John's wort, like vitamins, as a dietary supplement. This means that it can be sold without meeting requirements for safety and effectiveness. Talk with your physician about all dietary supplements and other complementary or alternative therapies that you are using or thinking of using. Some medications may be adversely affected by St. John's wort and other herbal compounds.

Exercise Modalities

Poor balance (postural instability) is a common symptom of Parkinson's disease. Balance disorders can easily lead to falls and significant injury, such as a fractured hip or injured knee. Thus, it is important to find ways to decrease the likelihood of falls.

There has been a great deal of research done with elderly people to find effective fall prevention interventions. Participating in an exercise regimen is one such effective, preventive strategy. It helps strengthen the muscles that surround joints, which will then act as natural brace to help keep the joints from giving way. Regular exercise also helps to maintain muscle mass. Forms of exercises that are highly recommended include taking daily walks, swimming, or bicycling on a regular basis. In addition to muscle strengthening, it is possible that, for people with Parkinson's disease, some types of exercise are better than other types. Specifically, some types may not only improve general physical fitness and muscle strength but may also improve balance and thus decrease the risk of falling.

Studies comparing Chinese exercise modalities to aerobic exercise training may help to identify exercise programs that are helpful in improving one's balance. Tai chi is an increasingly popular exercise in the United States and around the world. It is an ancient Chinese martial art in which slow, graceful movements of the body are coordinated with measured breathing. It is said to enhance balance, flexibility, cardiovascular fitness, and relaxation. It has also been shown to decrease falls and increase confidence in the elderly. Researchers in Sydney, Australia compared the number of falls in 702 essentially healthy men and women, over the age of sixty, who were either given lessons in Tai chi or not given any lesson at all (Voukelatos et al. 2007, 1185). The researchers found that the Tai chi participants decreased their risk of falling and improved their balance, as tested in a clinical laboratory.

A recent pilot study reported that Tai chi improved the ability to initiate walking and walk quickly in a small group of people with Parkinson's disease. This result is intriguing but must be studied in a larger group of people with Parkinson's disease. In addition, the pilot study did not look specifically at balance. To study the potential benefit of Tai chi in those with Parkinson's disease, NIH began recruiting people with Parkinson's disease to participate in a study comparing Tai chi and walk-run types of exercise. If it turns out that the people in the group doing standard aerobic exercise perform better on tests of balance, then the researchers will assume that the major benefit to Parkinson's disease patients comes from the building of muscle strength. If people in the Tai chi group do as well or better than the aerobic exercise group, this will suggest that there is another mechanism at work, perhaps a change to the motor control system of the brain. At the time of publication of this book, the results of this larger trial were not available.

In summary, there is a small body of evidence that indicates that complimentary therapies may be helpful for some people but not for everyone. In contrast, there is no evidence to support the use of alternative therapies in the treatment of Parkinson's disease. Thus, people with Parkinson's disease should take the medication prescribed by their neurologist so that they can move more easily and safely. Should one decide to use complementary therapies as well, it is important to remember that some complementary therapies may damage one's overall health. A big concern among doctors is that most patients do not tell them about the complementary therapies that they are using. Regardless of whether one has Parkinson's disease, another chronic illness, or is healthy, it is of utmost importance that one's doctor is aware of all the medications that are taken. That way, potential complications from the interactions between traditional prescription medication and complementary treatments can be avoided. Maintaining good health requires the establishment and maintenance of an honest, open dialogue between the patient and physician.

7

How Parkinson's Disease Affects the Family

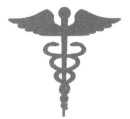

Michael J. Fox, the well-known actor, was diagnosed with Parkinson's disease at the age of thirty. At that time, he had young children who have since grown up with their father's illness. Instead of being afraid or upset by their father's tremor, Michael reports that he has turned it into a game for them. When the tremor is particularly prominent, his children sit on his lap and shout "go shaky, dad!" (taken from www.PR-inside.com, reported on Oct. 1, 2007)

P arkinson's disease, like any chronic illness, affects the entire family. For the adult child of someone with Parkinson's disease, it can signal the change in the parent-child relationship. The child, who is now an adult, is still accustomed to being the one who is cared for. Suddenly, that child becomes responsible for helping their parent. For teenagers who may have a parent or grandparent with Parkinson's disease, it can be particularly difficult. A teenager may be scared that they are going to develop Parkinson's disease or be embarrassed by the visible symptoms of the disease and try to ignore it and the affected family member.

Most people who have a chronic disease or are close to someone with a chronic disease experience some psychological distress. Many do not seek support from professional sources, feeling that they should not complain because the person with the disease is suffering far more than they are. The psychological challenges associated with chronic disease include obtaining and following through on medical treatment and advice, coping with emotional reactions such as depression and fear, and handling the impact of the disease on one's friends, relatives, and colleagues.

It is important to remember that anyone who is having trouble coping with the impact of a chronic disease should seek help. The help can come from many sources, including a supportive friend, teacher, clergy member, or professional counselor. Different people use different coping mechanisms when they are in stressful situations and to deal with "life" in general. Below are descriptions of some different coping styles that are used by most people.

COPING SKILLS

Direct problem solvers are individuals who go out to get answers and find support. Distancers are those who try to detach themselves from a problem. They refuse to think or do anything about a problem that is "staring them in the face." Positive thinkers are those who try to look at every problem as a growth experience. At the other extreme are the avoiders and the escapers. Avoiders engage in wishful thinking, "I hope that it will get better." Escapers may become involved in self-destructive behaviors, such as using alcohol or drugs.

Below are some case studies about people who had trouble coping with a friend or family member who had Parkinson's disease and examples of the coping strategies that helped them.

Ken

Ken is thirteen years old. For as long as he can remember, he has spent Sunday afternoons with his grandfather. His grandfather, whom he calls Papa Bobby, is seventy-five years old and has Parkinson's disease. Papa Bobby was diagnosed with Parkinson's disease five years ago, when he and his wife noticed that he was "slowing down" and had a tremor in his hand while watching television at night. Papa Bobby takes medication, but it doesn't work as well as it once did. Now, even with medication, his arms have a tendency to shake and he tends to "shuffle" when he walks.

Ken and Papa Bobby used to go for a walk every Sunday afternoon. They would go a block down the street, to the local ice cream parlor, to sit down and chat while eating their favorite Rocky Road ice cream with chocolate sauce. Lately, however, Ken has been refusing to go for walks. Ken prefers to spend Sunday afternoon in the house, watching television. Ken feels embarrassed by Papa Bobby's slow, shuffling gait. He is old enough to realize that most elderly people do not walk that way, and he is afraid that his friends will make fun of him if they see how his grandfather walks.

At first, Papa Bobby just assumed that the change in Ken's behavior was because he was a teenager. One day, however, Ken got into an argument with Papa Bobby and told him that he did not want his friends to see the two of them together. Papa Bobby was surprised, and hurt, and discussed the incident with his minister, Rev. Mathias. Because Ken attended the same church as Papa Bobby, Rev. Mathias decided to talk to Ken, to figure out what the underlying problem could be. When Ken and Rev. Mathias sat down to talk, Ken told him that he felt awful about what he had said to his grandfather. However, he then told him about his concern that friends would tease him and his own fear that he would "look like Papa Bobby" when he got old. After a long talk with Rev. Mathias and another long talk with Papa Bobby, Ken began to understand more about Parkinson's disease and how it affected his grandfather. Ken and Papa Bobby resumed their Sunday routine of walking down to the ice cream parlor together.

In this case study, Ken tried to cope with the problem by distancing himself, by refusing to spend as much time with grandfather as he used to. Fortunately, he was able to talk to his minister and then learned more about Parkinson's disease. Armed with this information, he returned to spending his Sundays with his grandfather.

Emma

Emma went to college and got a degree in civil engineering. She decided to move back to her hometown and accepted an exciting job with an architectural firm. Emma left for college five years earlier and had been home only for brief vacations. She and her parents agreed that she would move back into the family house for a short time, to save money for a down payment for a condominium of her own. The plan was that she would stay at home for a year, saving as much money as possible, and then find her own place.

Soon, Emma realized that something was seriously wrong with her dad, John. John had always been very active around the house and community. Now Emma noticed that he stayed home a lot. Sometimes, when they were watching a baseball game on television, she noticed that his right arm would shake. Emma convinced her dad that he needed to see a doctor. The family doctor examined him and made a tentative diagnosis of Parkinson's disease. However, the doctor also sent John to a neurologist to be certain of the diagnosis and to start treatment.

Emma accompanied her dad to the neurologist's office. When the doctor confirmed the diagnosis of Parkinson's disease, Emma was panic stricken. How could her dad, who took care of everything and was supposed to help her fix up her new condominium, be sick? What would happen to Emma, and what would happen to her mother and younger brother, Sean, who was still in high school? Emma decided that she would abandon her plans to move out. She would continue to live at home and help her parents cope with her dad's illness and help them to raise her younger brother.

John, however, handled the new of his diagnosis pretty well. He started taking the medication prescribed by the neurologist and felt much better. He started working in the yard again and took care of a couple projects around the house that he had abandoned.

In the meantime, Emma spent hours on the Internet trying to learn all that she could about Parkinson's disease. She was thrilled to learn that people with Parkinson's disease are able to live independently for many years. Emma started to attend a support group, sponsored by the American Parkinson's Disease Association, where she got to see and talk to other people with Parkinson's disease and their families. After talking to them and seeing how well her dad was doing on his medications, she realized that she could move out of the house, after all. The following year, as planned, she started looking for her own place to live.

Emma displays the traits of a direct problem solver. She got information from the Internet and support from others with Parkinson's disease. Armed with this knowledge, she was able to march on with her own independent, adult life.

Gabriel

Gabriel was sixteen years old when his dad was diagnosed with Parkinson's disease. At that time, Gabriel was so busy worrying about taking the SAT college entrance exam and applying to college that he did not think about his dad's health problems at all. In college, Gabriel decided to major in biology. In one class, he started to learn about Parkinson's disease and other neurological disorders. At the end of that semester, when he went home, he started to pay attention to how his father walked and began to notice his father's tremor. Gabriel started to worry about his dad. Gabriel started to read more about Parkinson's disease and began talking to his dad about the symptoms he had and what he did to overcome them. Gabriel soon became adept at discussing the risks and benefits of different anti-Parkinson medications, and he began to read about other neurological diseases as well. The more Gabriel learned, the more he became interested in the brain. In his senior year of college, he conducted a *research project in the neurobiology department. Based on his experience and interests, he decided to go to graduate school in neurobiology.*

Gabriel's story is an example of positive thinking, turned into positive action. Gabriel's academic interests and concern for his father merged into a career path that will allow Gabriel to make his own scientific contribution to our understanding of the brain.

Jasmin

Jasmin is twenty-four years old and just found out that her grandmother, with whom she grew up, has Parkinson's disease. Her grandmother managed to keep the news from her for more than a year. It was only when Jasmin noticed the medication in her grandmother's medicine cabinet that she was told her grandmother's diagnosis. Jasmin was shocked. She was also hurt that her grandmother, who meant the world to her, did not tell her about the illness right away. Jasmin did not know how to broach the topic with her grandmother, and so she did not bring it up at all. Gradually, Jasmin decided that Parkinson's disease must not be that serious, because her grandmother never talked about it.

Jasmin decided that the illness was not a big deal. She did not spend any time or effort in learning about the disease. Whenever she saw her grandmother, she would get upset to watch her arms shaking. Jasmin began spending more time with her friends and less with her family. Then, one day, she received a phone call from her uncle, telling her that her grandmother had died. Jasmin felt awful. She missed her grandmother and felt terribly guilty because she had not talked to or seen her for three months.

Clearly, using avoidance or escape coping mechanisms are not beneficial. In the case of Jasmin, it robbed her of precious time that she could have spent with her grandmother. There is some evidence that trying to avoid a problem creates an increased risk for psychological stress either in the short term or many years later in life. Better psychological outcomes have been associated with coping mechanisms that use positive thoughts and direct problem-solving behavior.

Jack and Nancy

Jack and his wife are fifty-eight years old. They were high school sweethearts and got married as soon as they both finished college. They worked as elementary school teachers and retired one year ago. They have two daughters, who are adults working and living on their own. Jack and Nancy had planned to go on an around-the-world trip the year after they retired.

In the months before retiring, Nancy noticed a "shaking" in her left hand. She assumed that it was caused by the stress of retiring and ignored it. Once she retired, she had more time to devote to her hobbies: knitting and making scrapbooks. The tremor in her left hand became more noticeable. She also started to have trouble when she was knitting; she could not make the knitting needle that was in her left hand move as easily as it had in the past. At first she thought it was arthritis. She started taking aspirin every day. However, her left hand did not get any better. She went to her doctor, Dr. Conseco, who noticed a rest tremor of the left arm. Dr. Conseco also noticed that her left arm did not move very much when she walked. After talking about the possibility that she has Parkinson's disease, Dr. Conseco referred her to a neurologist.

Nancy was visibly upset when she returned home. She talked to Jack, who told her not to worry. "You can't have Parkinson's disease," he kept saying. In fact, he was so certain that this was all a mistake that he refused to accompany her to the neurologist's office. So, Nancy went alone for an evaluation. The neurologist agreed that she may have Parkinson's disease and explained that it was necessary to monitor her and see how she responded to treatment.

When Nancy returned home from the neurologist's visit, she had a prescription in her hand and told her husband that the "doctor thinks it's Parkinson's disease." Jack refused to believe it. He went ahead and made their reservations for a trip to Italy, despite Nancy's misgivings about traveling now that she had started a new medication. "You're fine," Jack insisted. He told her not to fill the prescription. He was certain that the tremor would go away, once they were relaxed and on vacation.

Jack is trying to cope with Nancy's health problems by escaping them. Although this coping mechanism may work for a short period of time, it is not likely to help Jack in the future, once he returns from his trip and has to face Nancy and her persistent tremor.

WHEN IN-HOME HELP OR SKILLED NURSING CARE IS REQUIRED

One of the most difficult decisions that families and patients face, and often try to avoid, is what to do if independent living becomes difficult. The first concern may be over someone's ability to drive.

Having a diagnosis of Parkinson's disease does not, in and of itself, mean that a person must give up the car keys and never drive again. Keep in mind that the symptoms and severity of Parkinson's disease vary tremendously from one person to another. The biggest concern regarding driving centers on whether the reaction time of a person with Parkinson's disease is fast enough. Because one of the primary symptoms of Parkinson's disease is bradykinesia (slowness in movement), the concern is about the ability to hit the brake or steer quickly in an emergency.

Laws about who may and may not drive vary from state to state and can be found by contacting the local office of the Motor Vehicle Department. Most states have programs for evaluating drivers to determine who can drive safely. Some rehabilitation hospitals and clinics offer programs to evaluate a person's ability to drive as well.

In addition to difficulty with driving, as a person ages it is common that their ability to perform physical chores around the house becomes limited. Shoveling the driveway or mopping the floors, for example, require more physical agility than an eighty year old with Parkinson's disease may have. On a practical level, housekeeping services are typically available in large metropolitan areas and include assistance with house cleaning, cooking, and running errands. Although these services are not covered by insurance, they do extend the length of time that someone can live in their own home and so are worth the expense for those who can afford it.

A good place to start, to find services in a particular community, is to contact the local visiting nurses association (VNA). The VNA is a nonprofit agency that provides home healthcare for people of all ages and with any medical condition. To find the VNA in your area, check the local yellow pages or log onto the website for the Visiting Nurses Association of America (www.vnaa.org).

As a person ages and their disease progresses, it may become impossible to live independently even with housekeeping services. This typically occurs when a person needs help bathing and dressing and cannot prepare a meal independently. Even the most supportive family members or friends usually find it impossible to meet the physical and emotional demands of such a situation. This is the stage at which long-term arrangements in an extended care or nursing facility can become necessary.

Ideally, it is best if the person with Parkinson's disease addresses and plans for the possibility that assistance in daily living may be needed, makes plans in advance, and then discusses them in detail with family members and friends, years before the plan must be put into action.

There are many different types of assisted living facilities. The cost of these facilities varies as well, depending on what services are provided. Skilled nursing facilities provide nursing care twenty-four hours a day. Assisted living facilities typically provide separate apartments and a group dining area. It is up to the individual tenant whether to prepare their own meals or partake of the prepared meals in the dining room. In addition, different assisted living institutions provide different levels of available medical care, from weekly nursing visits to review one's medications to an on-call nurse, available twenty-four hours a day. A good resource for getting started is a publication from the National Institute on Aging. It is called *Long-Term Care: Choosing the Right Place* and is available at http://www.niapublications.org/engagepages/longterm.asp.

People who make these decisions and have them in place should the need arise could be saving partners and family members from a difficult task at a time of extreme stress and anxiety. For families in which the decision does have to be made in a hurry because their loved one is hospitalized, remember that the professionals in the hospital are skilled at facilitating these discussions and at helping you sort out feelings. Although people often feel that they are the only ones to have ever gone through this, they are not, and there are many people who can help.

Unfortunately, when children are involved in making the extended care or nursing home choices for an ill parent, it is altogether too common for old rivalries and bad feelings to emerge and interfere with decision making. This is usually extremely upsetting for families already under a great deal of stress. It may be helpful to know that doctors see the same fears and tensions in nearly every family and that advanced planning can help avoid conflicts. Here is a story that illustrates some of these issues.

John is seventy-five and has had Parkinson's disease for twenty years. His wife, Sally, is seventy-six and has limited mobility as a result of severe arthritis. They still live in the house where they raised their four children but only use the bottom floor because it's difficult for them both to climb the stairs.

Two of their children, Bill and Nancy, live nearby. Bill and Nancy are the two youngest children. The two older children, Jason and Richard, live 2,000 miles away. Jason comes home for the Christmas holidays and for a week in the summer. Richard, however, had a disagreement with his family about ten years ago and has not seen any of them since that time.

Bill and Nancy alternate taking days off from work to go with their parents to their numerous doctor appointments. They manage other aspects of their parents' lives, too. Nancy has arranged for lawn and housekeeping services for her parents and Bill takes care of all the house repairs. Bill and Nancy have had some discussions about what to do if one or both parents become "really sick," but neither has brought up the subject of putting them in an assisted living or nursing home.

John and Sally, whose own parents died at relatively young ages (all in their sixties), sometimes express disbelief that they have become as old as they are. They try to avoid discussions about the other's infirmities. They don't want to scare each other and insist that they are managing perfectly well.

Suddenly however, Sally has a massive heart attack and ends up in the intensive care unit of the local hospital. John, Bill, and Nancy maintain a constant vigil at the hospital. Jason manages to get on a plane and makes it to the hospital two days later. Unbeknownst to the siblings, John had also called Richard, urging him to come home to see his mother. One day later, Richard arrives at the hospital. Rather than stay with his father or siblings, he chooses to stay in a hotel. He talks to his dad and spends time in the hospital with his mother but does not speak to his siblings.

Sally survives the heart attack, but just barely. It is clear to the physicians, nurses, and physical therapists that care for her that she will require constant nursing care. The social worker, discharge coordinator, nurses, and physicians at the hospital have periodic discussions with John and the rest of the family regarding the best circumstances for Sally. Jason is quite shaken up and confides to his father and siblings that he believes that they are all being pressured to get Mom out of the hospital. He thinks that not everything that should have been done was done to treat Sally. Her mom did not have high blood pressure, she did not smoke, and there is no family history of heart attacks, so how could this have happened? Why didn't her regular physician pick up on some warning signs? And why is everyone giving up and sending Mom to a nursing home?

After spending a week at Sally's bedside, Jason finally realizes that his mom does, in fact, need constant care. He feels shocked and confused, but Bill and Nancy are less upset because they understood their mother's needs almost immediately. They also know that their dad is not healthy enough to care for Sally.

Jason, Bill, and Nancy try to talk to their estranged brother, Richard, about the situation. However, Richard continues to refuse to speak to them. Richard does speak to his dad, however, and tells his dad that mom needs more care than she can get at home. This conversation does help ease John's guilt about having to put his wife in a nursing facility.

Although everyone is unhappy about having to put Sally in a nursing facility, they all agree that it is the only choice. Nancy goes on a tour of several homes that the hospital discharge coordinator has recommended. All the facilities are close enough to her dad that he can take a bus to visit Sally every day.

This is a common situation, with some variations, of course, that can be found in many families. The divisions between the children cause significant tension and make it extremely difficult to come to an agreement regarding the placement of the parent. In the meantime, the hospital staff has completed its intensive treatment and evaluation of the patient. The insurance company is anxious to discharge the patient from the hospital, because she is not getting any treatment there that could not be provided in a skilled nursing facility, and the hospital administration, fearing that the insurance company will refuse to pay for additional days in the hospital, is anxious to have the family come to an agreement.

Help is available to aid in resolving situations like this. The family described above—to avoid a growing disagreement that they feared could lead to a family feud—participated in a series of meetings with the hospital staff. They talked with a hospital social worker and discharge planner on three separate occasions. They each, separately, talked with the hospital chaplain, too. Furthermore, there was a meeting with the physicians, nurses, and therapists who treated Sally. The emphasis was kept on what would be best for Sally based on the recommendations of the healthcare professionals who had no vested interest in the dynamics between the siblings or between them and their father. After these meetings and spending time talking together, all four children and their father finally agreed that Sally would be best served in a nursing facility that was close to home. With the assistance of the discharge coordinator at the hospital, they found a good facility and transferred Sally there.

There are several lessons to be learned from the experience of this family. One is how difficult it is to make a decision to change a living situation when declining health makes it necessary. Another is that even well-meaning and loving family members can complicate decision making because they may not fully understand the situation. Another is that hospitals have trained staff to aid in family conflict and decision making. The most important lesson is that it is helpful to think about, discuss, and plan for assisted living and nursing home arrangements long before they are needed.

8

Scientific and Clinical Research in Parkinson's Disease

A tremendous amount of research is being conducted to understand the cause of Parkinson's disease, its impact on people with the disease, and to develop better treatments. Research focusing on the cause of Parkinson's disease is referred to as basic scientific research. Research focusing on the impact of Parkinson's disease on every facet of a person's life is referred to as clinical research. Research focusing on the development of better treatments for Parkinson's disease is referred to as drug development. Both basic and clinical researches occur, primarily, at academic medical centers. The bulk of drug development research occurs in pharmaceutical companies.

Academic medical centers comprise a medical school and its associated hospital, where medical students, interns, and residents are trained. These centers have physicians, who treat those with Parkinson's disease and participate in clinical research, and scientists, who study the cause of Parkinson's disease. By working together, physicians and scientists have made enormous strides in improving treatments and understanding the pathology that underlies the changes seen in Parkinson's disease. Both NIH and several private foundations, including the Michael J. Fox and National Parkinson's Foundations, fund the basic science and the clinical research that are done on Parkinson's disease. The research itself is conducted at many levels, from genetic experiments that analyze DNA, to work in cells that share some of the features of brain cells and can be grown in a Petri dish, to work in rodents and nonhuman primates. The data obtained from these experiments are then synthesized to help direct pharmaceutical research that is aimed at developing better treatments for Parkinson's disease.

DNA experiments are done by molecular biologists. Molecular biology is the scientific discipline that focuses on DNA and how the genes we inherit influence our overall health. In Parkinson's disease research, molecular biologists and neurologists have worked closely together to identify the genes, and mutations in those genes, that cause Parkinson's disease in only a few families, as discussed in Chapter 3. The hope is that, by studying these genes, we will learn new information that will help everyone with Parkinson's disease, even those who do not have the particular gene mutation that is being studied.

Once molecular biologists and neurologists have finished their collaborative effort and a gene mutation has been identified, the next step is to understand how a gene mutation causes a disease. The simplest way in which to start these experiments is to study the effects of a gene mutation on a single cell. The advantage to working on single cells is that they are easy to manipulate. Scientists usually use cells that are easy to grow in a Petri dish but have some of the properties of the body organ that is affected by a particular disease.

In Parkinson's disease research, many scientists study cells that originally came from a brain tumor. The advantages of using brain tumor cells is that they grow quickly and have some of the characteristics that are found in healthy brain cells. The disadvantage of using these cells is that they are not from the substantia nigra, the region of the brain affected in Parkinson's disease, and they are isolated in a Petri dish. Cells grown in Petri dishes are referred to as being "in culture" and do not have connections or send messages to other brain cells. Thus, although doing experiments "in culture" can give important information about how proteins and specific mutations in proteins affect individual brain cells, it does not give any information about how proteins and specific mutations in proteins affect the way in which the entire brain functions. More work must be done, in animals, to understand the ways in which the entire brain is affected by a disease in which cells die in only one specific area within the brain.

The brain is a complex organ that cannot be thoroughly studied without the use of animal models. Within the brain, there are many different types of cells that perform distinct functions. The brain cells that help process language are very different from the cells that process visual information. Not only do these cells perform different functions, but they are found in completely separate regions of the brain and also look different. Different brain cells have marked differences in their appearance. The appearance of a cell is based on its shape and size and is referred to as its "morphology." For those scientists who study the brain, different cells can be identified by their appearance just as easily as someone else identifies friends by their appearance. In addition to the regional differences in the function and appearance of brain cells, they connect and transmit information to one another in an intricate web. If this web is disrupted, by injury or the death of cells in one specific brain region, the effects can be seen in the remote brain regions that were connected to the injured area.

As a comparison, let us consider that the connections between the different regions of the brain are similar to the connections made between airplanes, at various airports. Each airline has several airport "hubs," where many planes fly in and out to various cities. Each airport hub, where many airplanes congregate, is similar to the collection of brain cells that process language or visual information. Just as each plane that travels between them connects the airline hubs, the various collections of brain cells are connected by their axons that extend and send information to other brain regions. Just as a snowstorm in Chicago can disrupt any travel between the east and west coasts that requires changing planes at O'Hare airport, the loss of cells in one specific region of the brain affects the flow of information to other brain regions to which it is connected. Because these complex connections between brain cells cannot be reproduced in a test tube, it is essential to conduct research on brain diseases in animals.

Both NIH and local university committees govern all work involving animals to ensure that it is conducted in a responsible manner. Each university has an animal use committee, made up of veterinarians, scientists, and members of the community. The animal use committee reviews and must approve the details of all experiments involving animals or animal tissue before they can be performed. Once a scientist gets approval to conduct a specific series of experiments, he or she must then submit annual reports that detail the number of animals used and how they were treated. The animal use committee at each institution reviews these reports before giving permission for additional work to take place. In addition, agencies that fund scientific research will not release the funds to a scientist until he or she has gotten approval for any experiments that involve animals. There are many layers of oversight to ensure that animals are treated humanely and ethically and used only when necessary.

In addition to research to understand what happens in the brains of those with Parkinson's disease, clinical trials are conducted by both pharmaceutical companies and NIH to test medications or devices that may be of benefit to those with Parkinson's disease. The goal is to find which medication or treatment works best for a carefully defined group of people. Participants, also called study subjects, must meet strict criteria to enroll in a specific study. A research coordinator and doctor at a university, doctor's office, or clinic evaluate whether or not someone is eligible for the study that is being conducted. The subjects are not charged a fee to be part of a clinical trial. In fact, subjects are sometimes paid for their participation. NIH funds many of the medical trials in the United States. Below is a description of the methodology used in clinical research trials and the approval process that every potential new medication must go through before it is approved for use.

THE LONG ROAD TO MARKET

New drugs must be evaluated and approved by the FDA before they can be offered for sale. Clinical trials are an integral part of the evaluation process. The FDA requires that drugs go through three phases of clinical testing, with each phase involving progressively larger numbers of people who are tested over longer periods of time. A drug must be considered successful in each phase to move on to the next phase.

Phase 1 is to determine the metabolic and pharmacologic actions of a drug in humans and to determine possible side effects. The number of study subjects in a Phase 1 clinical trial is small, typically in the range of twenty to eighty subjects.

Phase 2 is to determine the safety and effectiveness of a drug. The number of study subjects varies from a few dozen to a few hundred.

Phase 3 is to determine the long-term benefits of the medication or device. The number of study subjects varies from a few hundred to a few thousand.

THE HISTORY OF THE FDA AND THE DRUG APPROVAL PROCESS

The FDA was given regulatory authority over the labeling and sale of drugs in 1906. However, it was not until 1938 that the United States Congress required that drugs obtain approval from the FDA before being sold. In the latter half of the twentieth century, a system of laboratory testing and human clinical trials was established to determine the safety and efficacy of the drugs that are sold in the United States.

Every potential drug is first analyzed in the laboratory. The physical and chemical properties of a drug are studied in a test tube. The pharmacologic and toxic effects of the drug are then tested in animals. If these results show promise, meaning that the drug helps in an animal model of a particular disease and does not cause significant toxicity, the company developing the drug can apply to the FDA to begin testing in humans. The FDA application, referred to as the Investigational New Drug Application (IND), must provide the data from the experiments done in test tubes and in animals, demonstrating that the drug may be beneficial and is not toxic. The IND must be reviewed and approved by the FDA before human clinical trials can begin.

Once the FDA gives approval for a particular drug to be tested in clinical trials, sites at which the drug will be tested must be established. Typically, clinical trial sites are established in academic medical centers where physicians and nurses who are skilled in treating people with the disease under study can serve as investigators. The investigators at each site are responsible for treating and monitoring the study subjects and reporting their findings to the FDA. Once each site and its local investigator are identified, permission to conduct the trial must also be gained from the institutional review board (IRB) of each site. Each academic hospital center has an IRB. The IRB is an independent body that includes physicians, nurses, and lay members of the community. The IRB reviews clinical research trials to ensure that they are run safely and fairly. The IRB is responsible for protecting the rights and welfare of subjects both before and during a clinical trial.

In a Phase 1 trial, only one or two sites may be established because relatively few subjects are required. However, Phase 3 trials require significantly more study subjects, and typically multiple sites (twenty or more) are established. In Phase 1 trials, a small number of healthy subjects are given the study drug. These studies assess the most common acute adverse effects and examine the size of the dose that people can take without the development of a high incidence of side effects. If Phase 1 studies do not reveal significant problems, then the drug proceeds to Phase 2 testing.

In Phase 2 trials, the study drug is given to those who have the disease that the drug is intended to treat. Researchers then assess whether the drug has a favorable effect on the condition. If results of Phase 2 studies are promising, then a large number of patients are recruited for Phase 3 trials.

Phase 3 trials are designed to assess safety, efficacy, and appropriate dosage of the study drug in those with the disease. The patients are treated with either the study drug or a placebo and are monitored for one to four years. A placebo is a pill that contains biologically inactive substances that is given to some persons who are participating in a study. The choice as to which subject gets placebo and which subject gets the active compound is made randomly. In well-designed clinical trials, neither the study subject nor the physicians evaluating the patient know who is getting what until the trial is completed and the results are analyzed. This type of clinical trial is referred to as "double-blind."

Once a Phase 3 trial is completed, a team of FDA physicians, statisticians, and pharmacologists review the data. Thus, the professionals who review the data do not work for the company developing the drug and do not have a financial stake in the company itself. If this independent and unbiased review establishes that the benefits of a drug outweigh its known risks, the drug is approved for sale.

It is very important to understand that participating in a clinical trial does not guarantee that one will receive the experimental drug. Some subjects will receive a placebo instead. Subjects are randomized to receive either the drug or the placebo. In most cases, the doctor, study staff, and subject will not know whether the active drug or the placebo was given until the study is over.

STUDIES OF THE HUMAN BRAIN

Another active area of research is the study of the human brain itself. Despite many of the advances described in this book, there is still a great deal about Parkinson's disease that is not understood. To advance our knowledge of Parkinson's disease, it is crucial to study the brains of those who had Parkinson's disease and compare them with the brains of those who died of other nonneurological causes. Many academic centers that focus on Parkinson's disease research also have brain donation programs for people who are interested and willing to donate their brain to research upon their death. The goal is that, by providing researchers with human brain tissue that can be studied in great detail, the knowledge obtained will improve the lives of future generations of people who will develop Parkinson's disease.

9

Case Studies in Parkinson's Disease

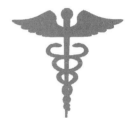

Below are a series of case studies that illustrate the ways in which Parkinson's disease may affect someone's life and how some of the symptoms can be alleviated with different medications. These case studies do not represent any specific person. Each is representative of the many different ways in which Parkinson's disease can affect an individual and his or her family.

BEN

Ben is seventy-four years old and was diagnosed with Parkinson's disease ten years ago. Ben takes carbidopa/levodopa (Sinemet) every three hours while he is awake. This translates into five or six tablets per day. When he first wakes up, Ben feels pretty slow and stiff. He keeps a glass of water and some medication on his nightstand, so that he can take a tablet as soon as he is awake. Then, he relaxes in bed for about half an hour. When he feels his feet and lower back start to loosen up, he gets out of bed and gets ready for the day.

Although Ben is retired, he remains fairly active. He plays golf three or four times a week. He also has a woodworking shop in his home. He likes to build furniture and tries to spend at least two hours a day in his shop. He usually works in the shop in the late morning, because this is the time of day when his ability to handle tools is at its best.

Lately, Sara, Ben's wife, has noticed that he "can't keep still" during dinner and throughout the evening. While they eat dinner, he sways back and forth in his chair. While they watch television, after dinner, his feet keep moving. Ben hasn't noticed these symptoms at all.

At his next visit with the neurologist, Sara goes along and tells the doctor what she has noticed. The doctor deduces that these symptoms are dyskinesias. The dyskinesias develop in the evening as the total amount of dopamine in Ben's brain has increased, thanks to the multiple doses of medication that he takes earlier in the day. To minimize the dyskinesias, the doctor recommends that Ben take the carbidopa/levodopa every four hours while awake, thereby reducing his total daily dose from six tablets, at the most, to four tablets.

Ben begins the new regimen and feels "lousy" within a few days. He finds that he has a harder time using the tools in his woodworking shop. His golf game has gotten worse. His average score has gone up by five strokes. However, Sara thinks that Ben is better. Ben does not move a lot in the evening. He doesn't move around in his chair during dinner. However, on the night that she made steak, she had to cut his for him because he had trouble handling the knife. While they watch television, Ben's feet remain still. However, she has noticed that his rest tremor has returned in the right arm. By the time they are ready to go to bed, Sara has to help Ben to stand up and he is already complaining that his forearm is sore.

After another week of feeling "lousy" on his new medication regimen, Ben calls the neurologist. When he goes in for another visit, it is clear to the doctor that Ben is more bradykinetic and rigid compared with his last neurological exam. After discussing his symptoms and educating Sara about the nature of dyskinesias, the doctor instructs Ben to resume taking his medication every three hours. Clearly, for Ben to remain mobile and pursue the hobbies that he enjoys, he needs more medication during the day. Because the dyskinesias are mild and not troubling for Ben, there is no need to try to minimize them.

MELINA

Melina is sixty-four years old and was diagnosed with Parkinson's disease seven years ago. At the time of her diagnosis, she had a rest tremor in her left hand and had trouble using her left hand to put in earrings or apply makeup. For five years, her tremor was well controlled with medication. During this time, she did slowly increase the number of times that she took medication during the day, but she was able to get at last two and a half hours of good tremor control with every dose of medication.

Over the past two years, however, her response to the medication has really changed. Now, thirty minutes after every dose of medication, she has uncontrolled movements of her arms and trunk that last for about twenty minutes. During this time, she cannot hold anything in her hands because she will drop it. Once these excessive movements subside, she has about sixty minutes when she is "good," meaning that she is not too stiff nor is she moving uncontrollably. It is during this sixty minute period that she tries to take care of her daily chores, such as showering and getting dressed or cooking dinner.

As soon as the hour is over, however, she feels her body "slow down." Her rest tremor returns, she becomes stiff, and she has trouble walking to a chair. She keeps medication with her all the time. She has learned to swallow her pills without needing any water. Her neurologist has also prescribed a new form of carbidopa/levodopa that disintegrates as soon as she puts it under her tongue. She manages to walk, although slowly and with a shuffling step, to her chair. She sits down, takes her next tablet, and waits for it to "kick in" so that she can perform the next set of chores.

Melina and her neurologist have been talking about treatment with DBS. The neurologist thinks that Melina is a good candidate, but she has been scared about undergoing brain surgery. Now, however, Melina is frustrated and would like to have more control of her movements for a longer period of time during the day. The doctor refers her to a movement disorders center, where hundreds of people have been treated with DBS. After the surgery, Melina spends a year making visits to the center every three months. During these visits, her stimulator settings are adjusted to give her maximum mobility.

Melina then returns to the care of her local neurologist. She takes medication only four times a day now, does not have any dyskinesias, and is able to move more easily throughout the day. She is quite happy that she underwent the surgery and feels more confident about her ability to live independently as she grows older.

EDUARDO

Eduardo is fifty-six years old and works as an attorney. For the last six months, his right hand and forearm have felt stiff and sore. Eduardo spends a lot of time typing on a computer keyboard. He was concerned that he had carpal tunnel syndrome. Eduardo went to his primary care doctor, who sent him for tests to determine whether he had carpal tunnel syndrome. The test came back negative. In the meantime, Eduardo made a conscious effort to cut back on the time he spent at his keyboard. This did not seem to have any effect on the soreness and stiffness that he felt in his right arm.

Over the next year, Eduardo noticed that his right hand tended to shake when he laid it on his desk. He also began to have trouble buttoning his shirt and tying his shoelaces. In addition, his secretary began to complain that his handwriting was hard to read. She worked for Eduardo for five years and did not have difficulty reading his writing until the six months before the day she discussed it with him. At this point, Eduardo realized that there must be something, other than carpal tunnel syndrome, that was affecting his right arm. He returned to his primary care doctor.

After examining him, Eduardo's doctor thought that he might have Parkinson's disease. He discussed this possibility with Eduardo and referred him to a neurologist for evaluation. The neurologist, Dr. Shah, also thought that Eduardo might have Parkinson's disease. Dr. Shah gave him a prescription for a dopamine agonist, ropinirole, and asked him to come back in three months. Eduardo felt much better after taking the medication for two weeks. His tremor did not appear at all during the day. He only noticed the tremor late at night, when he was tired, or when he was under stress. He was able to button his shirts without difficulty, but his secretary continued to complain about his handwriting!

Over the next two years, Eduardo continued to see Dr. Shah once every six months. Eduardo noticed that the tremor was "coming back" during the day. They increased his ropinirole (Requip) dose, and the tremor was controlled once again. Eduardo continued to respond to treatment and did not show any signs of dementia, visual hallucinations, rapid changes in heart rate or blood pressure, or the onset of frequent falls. Based on the lack of these features, his positive response to dopamine therapy, and his neurological exam, Dr. Shah confirmed the diagnosis of Parkinson's disease. He continued to treat Eduardo, who continued to work as an attorney without significant difficulty.

KAMLA

Kamla is seventy-five years old and lives alone, in her own apartment. She was a fifth grade teacher for many years and retired when she turned sixty-five. For the last ten years, she has been active by volunteering at her local temple, delivering meals to the homebound with Meals-on-Wheels, and teaching adults to read in a literacy class held at the local library.

Although Kamla lives alone, her nephew lives nearby. Her nephew is forty years old, and his name is Sanjeev. Sanjeev keeps a careful watch on his Aunt Kamla. Lately, Sanjeev has noticed that her voice has become softer and she is more difficult to understand when they speak on the telephone. Also, when he goes to her apartment for dinner, he has noticed that she walks more slowly from one room to another. She has trouble stirring pots on the stove and using silverware when they eat. One evening, Kamla tripped on a throw rug in her hallway. If Sanjeev had not been there to grab her, she would have fallen on the floor.

The near fall scared Kamla, and she talked to her doctor about it. Her doctor noticed some rigidity in her arms. He also saw that she took small, shuffling steps and her voice had become softer. Her doctor suspected that she had Parkinson's disease and began to treat her with carbidopa/levodopa. He also referred her to a local neurologist.

After a few weeks on the new medication, Kamla was able to walk more easily. She was able to chop vegetables, stir pots, and handle silverware as easily as she had one year before! However, her nephew and friends still had trouble understanding her on the telephone.

She discussed all of these symptoms, as well as her response to the carbidopa/levodopa, with the neurologist, Dr. Stevens. Dr. Stevens agreed, based on her response to dopamine replacement and the mild rigidity she detected on exam, that Kamla probably had Parkinson's disease. To help with her speech difficulty, Dr. Stevens referred her to a speech therapist. After undergoing intensive speech therapy, Kamla's voice was louder and clearer.

Although the medication helped significantly, Kamla was still afraid that she would fall. She underwent physical therapy, with an emphasis on walking and turning safely. She removed all the area rugs from her apartment so that she would not trip over them. She also had a special grab bar installed in her bathtub. A grab bar is a handle that is securely fastened to the studs that are behind a wall. A properly installed grab bar is strong enough to hold the weight of an adult and can help prevent a fall in the bathtub or shower. It is important to understand that a grab bar is very different from a towel rack. A towel rack is designed to hold the weight of a few towels only and is not securely fastened to the structural elements of the house (i.e., the wall studs).

SOPHIA

Sophia is eighty-two years old. She was diagnosed with Parkinson's disease fifteen years ago. She has never had a rest tremor but is slow and stiff in her movements. She also has trouble swallowing. She noticed that she was choking when she ate but did not tell anyone. Sophia lives in her own home alone and is afraid of being forced to live in a nursing home. As a result, she tries to ignore any changes in her health.

One year later, at the age of eighty-three, Sophia began to feel weak. Her skin felt clammy, and she was not able to get out of bed one morning. She dialed 911 and an ambulance transported her to the local emergency room. She was admitted to the hospital with a diagnosis of aspiration pneumonia. Her doctors suspected that the aspiration pneumonia developed because of underlying dysphagia. While in the hospital, Sophia had a swallow evaluation that revealed that her chewing was normal, but some of the food was ending up in her lungs rather than her stomach.

From the hospital, Sophia went to a rehabilitation facility for three weeks. At first, Sophia wanted to go home from the hospital. However, she knew that she was still fairly weak and so finally agreed to the transfer. At the rehabilitation facility, Sophia underwent physical, occupational, and speech therapy. Physical therapy helped to improve her strength and endurance. Occupational therapy helped her identify some gadgets that would help her at home, such as a long-handled shoehorn. In speech therapy, she learned techniques to help her swallow her food properly. At the end of her stay, Sophia felt confident that she could take care of herself at home.

To ease her transition back to her house, she also agreed to periodic checks by a visiting nurse. Each community has a nonprofit VNA. The VNA provides home healthcare to people of all ages, with any type of medical condition. When Sophia returned to her home, a nurse from the VNA checked on her three days a week to ensure that she was taking the proper pills at the proper time and that she was truly able to care for herself. It was soon clear that Sophia was perfectly independent, and the VNA services were terminated.

ALEC

People in the early stages of Parkinson's disease are typically able to work and travel without too much difficulty, provided that they remember to take their medication with them. If travel involves going to different time zones, there may be some difficulty and confusion in adjusting the time at which the medication should be taken. Here is an example of how someone may make these adjustments.

Alec is fifty-nine years old and was diagnosed with Parkinson's disease four years ago. Alec lives in New York and is planning a trip to London to visit some friends. He takes one tablet of carbidopa/levodopa four times a day and is not sure how to adjust this on the day of his flight. He spoke to his neurologist, who made the following recommendations.

On the day of his departure, his flight will leave New York at 6:30 P.M. and reach London at 6:30 A.M., local time, which is 1:30 A.M. in New York. Therefore, as far as Alec's brain and body are concerned, it will be 1:30 A.M. when he lands in London. On the day of the trip and while on the plane, Alec will take his medication at the usual scheduled time and keep his watch on New York time to do so. About forty-five minutes before the plane lands in London, Alec will take one additional tablet of carbidopa/levodopa. This extra pill will kick in just as the plane has landed and the passengers are allowed to leave the plane. This will allow him to walk and handle his passport and other travel documents more easily after he gets off the plane. Remember that the medications used to treat Parkinson's disease do not affect the course of the disease. Thus, taking one additional pill on occasion will not have any long-term negative effects on the disease. After Alec collects his bags, goes through customs, and reaches his hotel, he immediately takes a nap. Once he wakes up, it will be late morning or early afternoon in London. At that time, he will resume his usual medication regimen, using the local time to determine when to take the next dose.

JUNIOR HIGH SCHOOL DANCE

Monica was thirteen years old and about to attend her first school dance. Her grandmother, Marta, was active in the parent-teacher's association and had volunteered to serve as a chaperone. Monica was mortified by the fact that her grandmother would be at the dance. Her mom could not understand why she was so upset, because the mothers of two of her friends were also acting as chaperones.

Monica was worried that her friends would see how her grandmother's hands shook and see that it was hard for her grandmother to walk. Monica was afraid that her friends would not want to come to her house or talk with her at school if they saw that her grandmother was ill. Monica could not talk to her mother about this, because she knew that she should not feel this way. Not only was Monica embarrassed by the thought of everyone at school finding out about her grandmother's illness, but she also felt guilty about the fact that her grandmother's condition embarrassed her. Monica loved her grandmother dearly but saw her school friends as being part of a different world. Monica wanted to keep these two worlds separate.

On the day of the school dance, Monica began to complain of a stomachache. She told her mom that she could not go to the dance because she felt awful. Her mom was surprised and began to suspect that something else was going on, because Monica had eaten well earlier that day and rarely got sick.

Monica did not want to talk to her mom, however, and went to her room and closed the door. An hour later, her grandmother came over to take her to the dance. Her grandmother went into her room, to find out what was wrong.

She found Monica lying on her bed, crying. Finally, because she had never kept secrets from her grandmother, Marta told her that she was afraid that her friends would no longer be her friends if they saw how sick her grandmother was. Marta was surprised to hear this because she continued to live independently and was active in the school as well as in her local church. However, Marta started to talk about what her doctor had told her about Parkinson's disease. Marta told her granddaughter that no one knows why some people get Parkinson's disease and others do not. It is not an illness that can be "passed on," like a cold or the flu, from one person to another. So, if Monica's friends became afraid to come to her house or be near her out of fear, this would be the perfect opportunity for Monica to teach them about Parkinson's disease.

Marta went on to talk about the symptoms that she did have: the shaking of her arms, the fact that it took her longer to go on her daily walks than it used to, her trouble with putting on makeup. She also talked about all the things that she was able to do, thanks to the medications that her neurologist prescribed: live on her own, cook and bake for her family, volunteer at the school and at her church. The more that Marta talked about what she could do and the more information she gave her granddaughter about Parkinson's disease, the calmer Monica felt. As her grandmother urged, if her friends were mean to her or stopped being so friendly. then she should educate these so-called friends about Parkinson's disease and then find new friends!

By the end of the conversation, Monica felt better and had also learned quite a bit about Parkinson's disease. She and her grandmother never had a conversation about it before. Monica had no idea that her grandmother's symptoms could and were being controlled with medication. Monica had no idea that Parkinson's disease was not an illness that could be passed from one person to the next. The more information Monica got, from talking frankly with her grandmother, the better she felt. She was then able to attend the dance, with her grandmother acting as a chaperone, and was happy and relieved that no one asked her why her grandmother's hands were shaking.

Special events such as school graduations are joyous occasions that parents and children like to celebrate together. At these times, we expect our family members to share in the happiness of the occasion and celebrate with us. However, what happens if one parent has a chronic illness, making it difficult for them to reliably participate in an important family event? The following stories demonstrate how some families coping with Parkinson's disease work together to overcome these challenges.

SCHOOL GRADUATION

Tuesday, June 10: four days until high school graduation. Jim was relaxing at home now that his last round of high school final exams was over. Jim and his fellow seniors had a few days to relax and have fun before their graduation ceremony on Saturday. In the fall, Jim would head to New York University. He was really excited about living away from home and about being in the heart of New York City!

Jim is the eldest of three children. Everyone in his family is very excited about Jim's future. His younger brother cannot wait until the fall, when he will move into Jim's room. His parents and grandparents are looking forward to the ceremony itself. Ed, Jim's dad, is both excited and very worried that his symptoms of Parkinson's disease will interfere with his ability to enjoy his son's graduation.

Ed is fifty-seven years old and was diagnosed with Parkinson's disease two years ago. At that time, he noticed a sense of stiffness in his right arm that he thought was a strained muscle. At first, Ed ignored it and then tried to treat it with a heating pad and massages. Six months later, the stiff sensation became more bothersome. Ed started to notice that he had difficulty typing on a computer keyboard, his fingers were slower in their action, and he was making more mistakes when he typed. He saw a neurologist, who suspected that he had Parkinson's disease and prescribed the dopamine agonist ropinirole (Requip). After taking the medication for six weeks, during which time he slowly increased the dose according to his doctor's instructions, Jim could notice a marked difference in his symptoms. The stiff sensation in his arm was gone, and his typing skills improved. He was not as good at typing as he had been when he was younger, but he was definitely better than he had been before he started to take ropinirole (Requip). He now takes ropinirole (Requip) three times a day, and his symptoms are well controlled. He only feels a sensation of stiffness in his right arm and has difficulty using the fingers of his right arm if he forgets to take a dose of medication or if he is under stress or feeling ill.

Because Ed knows that he will be excited and anxious on the day of his son's graduation, he is afraid that he will not be able to drive everyone to the auditorium where the ceremony will be held. He is also concerned that he will not be able to take pictures of the event. Since their first child was born, Ed has been the family photographer. He wants to get good pictures of his son's graduation but is reluctant to give up this responsibility to others. To Ed, giving up his role as family photographer is a concession to the fact that he has Parkinson's disease, and he is afraid that, once he gives up on performing one activity, his ability to perform other tasks will be lost as well. As far as Ed was concerned, he had to make one of two unpalatable choices: give up on photography and admit that the Parkinson's disease was "taking over" or continue to take pictures and run the risk of not getting any clear, sharp pictures of Jim's graduation ceremony.

Ed talked the situation over with his wife, Mary. Fortunately, Mary used "positive thinking" frequently as a coping skill and had a knack for turning a situation from bleak to promising. In this particular case, Mary also knew something about their fifteen-year-old daughter Kate that Ed did not. Kate was developing an interest in photography and had taken a course in digital photography in her spring semester at school. Mary thought that this was the perfect opportunity to acknowledge Kate's growing maturity, by entrusting her with photography duties at her brother's graduation. In this way, Ed was not "giving up" on photography; he was passing it down to his daughter and would be able to transmit his interest in photography to her and watch her develop her own style and photographic interests.

WEDDING

Monday, September 2: five days before Jenna's wedding. She was busy running errands for the big day. Although the final head count for the reception had been given to the caterer and the band, photographer, and florist had all been confirmed, Jenna still had to pick gifts for her bridesmaids, shop for clothes for her honeymoon, and wrap the small picture frames that she and her fiancé had chosen to give to each guest. These minor errands were keeping her busy but not causing any stress. Jenna was feeling stressed and anxious about her dad.

Dad was sixty-four. Nine years ago, he was diagnosed with Parkinson's disease. Dad had a tremor and tended to walk by taking tiny steps, with his head down. At home, he had fallen backwards twice in the past two months while going up the stairs. All of his symptoms got worse when he was nervous. Jenna knew that, on the day of her wedding, her dad would be nervous, happy, and sad all at the same time. Although Jenna was ashamed to admit it, she was afraid that she would be embarrassed if her dad fell while walking her down the aisle.

Dad was worried about the walk down the aisle as well. He wanted, more than anything, to walk Jenna down the aisle without any difficulty. Fortunately, he had been planning for this day for the last three months. After Jenna had announced her engagement and chosen a date for the wedding, her dad had talked to his neurologist. They put together a plan that involved intensive physical therapy sessions in the weeks before the wedding.

By working with a physical therapist with a lot of experience in treating people with Parkinson's disease, dad was able to strengthen his leg muscles. He also put in a lot of hours, practicing to walk by putting each foot down carefully and completely with each step. Also, with the help of his neurologist, he was able to adjust the timing of his medication doses in the days before the wedding to ensure that the medication would be at its peak for the wedding ceremony.

In addition to walking down the aisle, Jenna and her dad want to have a perfect "father-daughter" dance at the reception. To help her dad do a simple two-step, Jenna chose a slow-tempo song with a prominent beat. In the months before the wedding, Jenna and her fiancé had taken dance classes. Jenna also got her dance instructor's help in working with her and her dad so that they could find a good song and simple dance to do together.

On the day of the wedding, Jenna and her dad were anxious, happy, and scared! While she was getting dressed, she thought back over the four years that she and her fiancé, Jon, had dated. Jon first asked her to marry him two years ago. At that time, Jenna said no and they had broken up for a few months. Jenna loved Jon but was determined to never marry. Jon was persistent, however, and once they resumed dating she told him why she said no. Jenna's grandfather and father had Parkinson's disease. Jenna had memories of her grandfather shuffling around the house and with a tremor that was so severe that her grandmother had to help him shave and get dressed. When her Dad was diagnosed with Parkinson's disease four years ago, she had been devastated. She was worried about her dad, of course, but also about herself. With two family members suffering from the same disease, she was convinced that she would get Parkinson's disease as well. Although she had always wanted to get married and have children, she decided that it would be better not to do so, because she did not want to have a child who was destined to develop Parkinson's disease.

Once she finally discussed these concerns with Jon, he was able to convince her to talk to a doctor about them. Jenna talked to her doctor, who advised her to see a genetic counselor. After both her doctor and the genetic counselor told her that the majority of cases of Parkinson's disease occur in people without a family history of the disease and that there is no way to test people for the disease before they have developed symptoms, Jenna realized that she should let go of her fear and live her life the way she had always wanted. Jon talked with the genetic counselor as well. Although Jon was not afraid that their children would develop Parkinson's disease, he decided that it would be good for both of them to learn about the illness and the risks associated with getting it. After they spent another year dating and talking endlessly about these and other issues, Jon proposed again and Jenna said yes.

Before she knew it, Jenna was fully dressed for the wedding. Her walk down the aisle with dad was flawless. At the reception, they danced without too much trouble. Her dad almost stumbled on the train of her gown, but he did not fall and they managed to finish the dance without any serious mishap. The next morning, Jenna and Jon left on their honeymoon while her dad stayed at home to pay the bills!

Resources

Thanks to the Internet, there is a plethora of sources for information about Parkinson's disease. It is important to choose sources of information carefully. Below are the names of several organizations that can help you learn more about Parkinson's disease. Some of the organizations listed below are geared toward scientists, physicians, and other professionals. Other organizations are dedicated to provide greater information and help to those with Parkinson's disease. Some of the organizations provide detailed scientific and medical information, whereas others provide practical information for people with Parkinson's disease, such as where to go for local nursing services.

The description about each resource is meant to give an overview regarding the services and mission that each particular agency, foundation, or website provides. In particular, information that comes from United States government organizations and from professional Parkinson's disease foundations is particularly well researched, thoughtful, and reliable.

If one is concerned about a particular friend or family member, then information gathering should include that person as well. Sharing knowledge is the best way to dispel fear and sort fact from myth. If the friend or family member permits, it is also helpful to discuss any topics that are of particular concern with the neurologist who is treating him or her.

Please note that phone numbers, street addresses, and website addresses are subject to change. The information provided here was accurate at the time that this book was published.

American Academy of Neurology (AAN)
www.aan.com
1080 Montreal Avenue
Saint Paul, MN 55116
Phone: (800) 879–1960 or (651) 695–2717

AAN is a professional society for medical specialists. The mission of AAN is to advance the art and science of neurology, thereby promoting the best possible care for people with neurological disorders. AAN offers professional development courses for physicians and other health professionals. AAN website also contains a section for the public, with links to other websites dedicated to neurological diseases.

American Neurological Association (ANA)
www.aneuro.org
5841 Cedar Lake Road
Suite 204
Minneapolis, MN 55416
Phone: (952) 545–6284

ANA is a professional society of academic neurologists and neuroscientists. The mission of ANA is to advance the goals of neurology, train and educate physicians in neurology, and expand the understanding of diseases of the nervous system and their treatment.

American Parkinson's Disease Association (APDA)
www.apdaparkinson.org
National office:
1250 Hylan Boulevard
Suite 4B
Staten Island, NY 10305–1946
Phone: (800) 223–2732 or (718) 981–8001
E-mail: apda@apdaparkinson.org
West Coast office:
10850 Wilshire Boulevard
Suite 730
Los Angeles, CA 90024–4319

Phone: (800) 908–2732 or (310) 474–5391
E-mail: apdawc@earthlink.net

APDA coordinates the operations of more than fifty chapters throughout the United States. APDA provides education, referrals for medical care, and counseling. It also raises funds to support research on the causes of and treatments for Parkinson's disease.

ClinicalTrials.gov
www.clinicaltrials.gov

This website provides information about ongoing clinical research trials. The site provides a list of research trials that are in progress and also information about the purpose of the research, the criteria for participation in the trial, and contact information for the persons running the trial.

Healthfinder
www.healthfinder.gov

Healthfinder is a useful website that contains health news, information about healthcare resources, and a library rich with information about health and medicine. Information about Parkinson's disease ranges from the general (overviews and descriptions of the disease) to the highly specialized (depression and Parkinson's disease, occupational therapy, and more). The Healthfinder project is coordinated by the Office of Disease Prevention and Health Promotion, which is part of the Department of Health and Human Services.

MedlinePlus
www.medlineplus.gov
www.nlm.nih.gov/medlineplus/parkinsonsdisease.html

MedlinePlus is a valuable health information website of the United States government. It is updated daily in English and Spanish, for health professionals and consumers, with facts and findings about a variety of health conditions. For every disease that is covered, the latest news and information about clinical and laboratory research, disease management, medications, nutrition, treatments, genetics, and legal matters are given. The Parkinson's disease section can be accessed at the website listed above.

Michael J. Fox Foundation for Parkinson's Research
www.michaeljfox.org
Church Street Station
P.O. Box 780

New York, NY 10008–0780
Phone: (800) 708–7644

The Michael J. Fox Foundation provides funding for research into the causes and cures for Parkinson's disease. One of the primary aims of this foundation is to increase the pace of discovery by raising funds to support innovative research.

Movement Disorder Society (MDS)
www.movementdisorders.org
555 East Wells Street
Suite 1100
Milwaukee, WI 53202–3823
Phone: (414) 276–2145
E-mail: info@movementdisorders.org

MDS is an international, professional society of clinicians and scientists who treat and conduct research on Parkinson's disease and other movement disorders. The mission of MDS is to disseminate knowledge about movement disorders, promote research into the causes, prevention, and treatment of movement disorders and to promote public policy that will support the care of patients with movement disorders.

National Center for Complementary and Alternative Medicine (NCCAM)
www.nccam.nih.gov

NCCAM is part of the National Institutes of Health. NCCAM supports research on complementary and alternative medicine and distributes information and advisories about complementary and alternative treatments.

National Institute of Neurological Disorders and Stroke (NINDS)
www.ninds.nih.gov

NINDS is part of the National Institutes of Health. NINDS funds research into a broad array of neurological disorders, including Parkinson's disease. A special section of the NINDS website describes the goal for Parkinson's disease research, which is to "ensure that extraordinary opportunities to move toward a cure are adequately supported and that critical obstacles to progress are addressed." The NINDS website contains valuable, up to date facts and information about research findings and treatment for Parkinson's disease.

National Parkinson Foundation (NPF)
www.parkinson.org

1501 NW 9th Avenue/Bob Hope Road
Miami, FL 33136–1494
Phone: (800) 327–4545

The goal of NPF is to find the cause of and cure for Parkinson's disease through research and to improve the quality of life for persons with Parkinson's disease. NPF also educates patients, caregivers, and the public about Parkinson's disease by sponsoring support groups, seminars, and publications.

The Parkinson Alliance
www.parkinsonalliance.net
P.O. Box 308
Kingston, NJ 08528–0308
Phone: (800) 579–8440 or (609) 688–0870

The Parkinson Alliance raises funds for pilot research projects. The goal is to provide the seed money to allow scientists to generate preliminary data that can be used to develop a large-scale research program, funded by the National Institutes of Health. The alliance is a nonprofit organization that channels 100 percent of the money it raises into research focused on Parkinson's disease.

Parkinson's Action Network (PAN)
www.parkinsonsaction.org
1025 Vermont Avenue, NW
Suite 1120
Washington, DC 20005
Phone: (800) 850–4726 or (202) 638–4101
E-mail: info@parkinsonsaction.org

PAN is a patient-advocacy group that works to increase government financial support of research on Parkinson's disease. PAN also works to ensure that people with Parkinson's disease have access to treatment for Parkinson's disease and that people with Parkinson's disease are not discriminated against in the workplace.

Parkinson's Disease Foundation (PDF)
www.pdf.org
1359 Broadway
Suite 1509
New York, NY 10018
E-mail: info@pdf.org

PDF seeks to help people with Parkinson's disease and their families. PDF provides information, sponsors professional and community conferences, awards research grants, and advocates for increased spending by the federal government for research into the causes and cure of Parkinson's disease.

PDTrials.org
www.pdtrials.org

This website was developed to increase patient participation in clinical trials. The site contains listings of clinical trials for the treatment of Parkinson's disease. The site also disseminates updates regarding Food and Drug Administration actions in approving and regulating those drugs that are used in the treatment of Parkinson's disease. The website was developed by a collaboration between numerous Parkinson's disease advocacy groups, including the Parkinson's Disease Foundation, the National Parkinson Foundation, the Michael J. Fox Foundation, and the National Institutes of Health.

Society for Neuroscience (SfN)
www.sfn.org
1121 14th Street, NW
Suite 1010
Washington, DC 20005
Phone: (202) 962–4000
E-mail: info@sfn.org

For those of you who are interested in neuroscience, which is the study of the nervous system, SfN is a good source of information. SfN is dedicated to advancing the understanding of the brain and nervous system. It is also committed to providing educational resources for undergraduates, graduate students, and scientists at all stages of their career.

Visiting Nurses Association of America (VNAA)
www.vnaa.org
Boston office:
99 Summer Street
Suite 1700
Boston, MA 02110
Phone: (617) 737–3200
E-mail: vnaa@vnaa.org
Washington office:
8403 Colesville Road

Suite 1550
Silver Spring, MD 20910–6374
Phone: (240) 485–1857
E-mail: vnaa@vnaa.org

VNAA is the national association of nonprofit, community-based home health organizations. Each local chapter is known as a visiting nurse association (VNA). Each VNA chapter is dedicated to bringing compassionate, high-quality and cost-effective home care to individuals in their community. To find out what in-home healthcare services are available in your community, go to the website listed above or find your local VNA in the yellow pages.

Worldwide Education and Awareness of Movement Disorders (WE MOVE)
www.wemove.org
204 West 84th Street
New York, NY 10024
E-mail: wemove@wemove.org

The WE MOVE organization runs an Internet site dedicated to the dissemination of knowledge about movement disorders for patients, doctors, and the general public. To learn more about Parkinson's disease and other disorders, this website offers excellent tutorials and video clips illustrating various movement disorders.

Timeline

175 AD   The prominent Greek physician Galen, who served as physician to prominent members of the Roman Imperial Court, describes the "shaking palsy" in his extensive medical texts.

1400   The ancient Indian medical text *Basavarajiyam* includes a description of Parkinson's disease. In Sanskrit, Parkinson's disease is referred to as Kampavata. Traditional Indian medicine used several natural products for the treatment of Parkinson's disease. One powdered seed, called *Atma gupta*, contains levodopa. Another seed, *Hyoscyamus niger*, has anti-cholinergic properties.

1817   Dr. James Parkinson published a treatise, *Essay on the Shaking Palsy*, describing six of his patients that appeared to have the same condition. The disorder was characterized by rigidity, rest tremor, stooped posture, and an accelerated gait.

1850s   The French neurologist Jean Martin Charcot observed and published more details regarding the disorder. Charcot described the full clinical spectrum of this disease and noted in depth the effects on the autonomic nervous system and the pain that can accompany the disease. Charcot was the first to suggest using the term "Parkinson's disease" for this disorder.

1888   The British physician Gowers, in his text "*Manual of Diseases of the Nervous System*," describes his personal experience with eighty patients from his London practice.

1920s   Anatomic studies of the brains of people who had Parkinson's disease reveal the pathologic abnormalities in the substantia nigra.

1961   Swedish and Austrian scientists identify that individuals with Parkinson's disease have dramatically lower levels of dopamine in the basal ganglia of their brains.

1960s   Scientists and physicians in Sweden, Austria, and the United States demonstrate that administration of levodopa improves the symptoms of Parkinson's disease.

1983   The American physician William Langston identified the toxin MPTP (1-methyl-4-phenyl-1,2,3,6-tetrahydropyridine) as causing an acute, permanent Parkinson-like state in those who inject it. This allowed scientists to use MPTP to create a variety of animal models of Parkinson's disease.

1987   Physicians at the University of Grenoble in France published the results of the use of deep brain stimulation for the treatment of Parkinson's disease.

Future We will be able to use gene therapy to stop or slow down the loss of dopamine-producing brain cells and use stem cells to replace the dead dopamine-producing brain cells and truly cure the disease.

Glossary

Acetylcholine: Acetylcholine is a chemical neurotransmitter that is released from the end of nerve fibers. It is involved in the regulation of essential functions of the body, such as heart rate and respiratory rate.

Activities of daily living: Activities of daily living are basic tasks of everyday life, such as eating, bathing, dressing, toileting, and transferring from bed to chair or chair to an upright position.

Akathisia: Akathisia is the term used to describe an inner sensation that a person has of having to move. It results in an inability to sit still.

Akinesia: Akinesia is a term used in neurology to refer to a lack of movement.

Amino acid: Amino acids are the building blocks of proteins.

Anhedonia: This term refers to the inability to derive pleasure from acts that normally provide pleasure to someone. It can be a symptom of depression.

Anosmia: This is the loss of the ability to smell.

Anticholinergic: An anticholinergic is a medication that blocks the action of acetylcholine. Two examples of anticholinergic drugs are trihexyphenidyl (Artane) and benztropine (Cogentin).

Anxiety: Anxiety is a heightened state of concern. Someone who is anxious might feel nervous or have a sinking feeling that something has gone, or is about to go, terribly wrong.

Apathy: Apathy refers to a lack of emotion or feeling.

Aphasia: Aphasia is an impairment in the ability to understand or utilize language.

Arthritis: Arthritis is a group of conditions in which there is damage to the joints of the body.

Aspiration: Aspiration is the inhalation of food or liquid into the airways or lungs rather than into the stomach. It can result in pneumonia.

Ataxia: Ataxia is the loss of balance as a result of a failure of the brain to coordinate movement. People who are ataxic appear wobbly and uncoordinated. The staggered gait of an intoxicated person can be described as ataxic.

Attention: This is the cognitive process of selectively concentrating on one aspect of the environment while ignoring everything else.

Autonomic nervous system: This is the subset of the nervous system that regulates the internal organs, without our conscious knowledge. For example, the autonomic nervous system regulates heart rate, respiratory rate, one's ability to perspire, the release of urine, and the diameter of the pupils.

Autosomal dominant: This is one of several ways in which a trait or disease is inherited in a family. An autosomal dominant disease is one in which only one copy of the disease-causing gene is required for the illness to develop.

Autosomal recessive: This is another way in which a trait or disease is inherited in a family. An autosomal recessive disease is that in which two copies of the disease-causing gene are required, one from the mother and one from the father, for the illness to develop.

Axon: This is a slender projection from the body of a nerve cell that transmits electrical impulses.

Ayurveda: Ayurvedic medicine is an ancient system of healthcare that is native to the Indian subcontinent. It promotes healthy living along with therapeutic measures that relate to physical, mental, social, and spiritual harmony.

Bipolar disorder: Bipolar disorder is a psychiatric condition characterized by episodes of depression alternating with episodes of mania.

Blepharospasm: Blepharospasm is the uncontrolled contraction of muscles of the face surrounding the eye. The eyelids close and can be difficult to open naturally.

Botulinum toxin: This is a protein produced by the organism *Clostridium botulinum*. It is a poisonous substance, when taken orally in large doses. In small doses, it is injected directly into muscle to treat dystonia.

Bradykinesia: This is another term for slowness of movement. Bradykinesia is one of the cardinal signs of Parkinson's disease.

Bradyphrenia: This is a term for the slowness of thought processes. It is similar to bradykinesia, in that bradykinesia refers to slowness of movement and bradyphrenia refers to slowness of thought.

Cachexia: This is a state of malnutrition.

Carbidopa: Carbidopa is a drug that is administered along with levodopa (L-dopa) to prevent L-dopa from being broken down before it enters the brain.

Cardinal signs: Parkinson's disease, like other disorders, is diagnosed through the display in a patient of cardinal signs. They are the most common signs exhibited by a majority of people with a disorder.

Carpal tunnel syndrome: This is a medical condition in which nerves become compressed in the wrist. It typically occurs in response to repetitive motion, such as typing. It leads to pain and weakness in the forearm and hand.

Cerebrovascular disease: A group of disorders in which the brain is transiently or permanently affected by a lack of oxygen or uncontrolled bleeding caused by a pathologic process that involves one or more of the blood vessels that supplies the brain.

Chorea: These are brief, irregular contractions of muscles in the hands or feet. They are not rhythmic and have a flowing, dance-like appearance.

Cognition: The mental processes that encompass all of the input and output of the brain. This includes activities such as using language and arithmetic during a trip to the grocery store, complex decision making such as selecting between two college admission offers, and the ability to understand things from another person's perspective.

Cognitive/behavioral therapy: A type of psychotherapy in which the goal is to modify everyday thoughts and behaviors to positively influence emotions.

Commode: Often used in nursing homes, it is a metal chair with a built-in container to hold urine and fecal waste.

Constipation: This term refers to infrequent bowel movements and/or the passing of hard stools or straining to have a bowel movement. In those with Parkinson's disease, constipation is thought to occur because the muscles of the colon contract too slowly, causing increased transit time for stool.

Cued recall: A form of memory, in which one can remember a specific fact when given information regarding that fact.

Deep brain stimulation: This is a technique in which electrodes are implanted in the brain to control symptoms of Parkinson's disease.

Delusion: A delusion is a false belief to which a person strongly adheres. Someone who was born and raised in the United States but thinks that he is the King of England, for example, is suffering from a delusion. This is called a grandiose delusion. There are also delusions of paranoia (of malicious plots) and somatic delusions (of illness). In Parkinson's disease, some patients develop delusions that can be related to medications.

Dementia: Dementia is an irreversible and progressive decline in a person's ability to form new memories, retrieve old memories, and perform complex tasks.

Depression: Depression is an illness characterized by excessive sadness, persistently low mood, or significant loss of pleasure and interest. It can usually be treated successfully with antidepressant medications. Depression is a common psychological event in Parkinson's disease.

Differentiation: The process by which an unspecialized cell becomes specialized into one of the many cell types that are found in the human body.

Diffuse Lewy body disease: This is one of the Parkinson's Plus syndrome diseases. People with diffuse Lewy body disease have some signs of parkinsonism, such as a rest tremor and/or rigidity. However, they also develop dementia that progressives relatively quickly, over one to three years, with frequent visual hallucinations.

Diuretic: A diuretic is a drug or other compound (e.g., coffee) that increases the production of urine.

Dopamine: Dopamine is a chemical neurotransmitter that is released at the end of nerve fibers and is essential for the proper functioning of the brain. Dopamine is deficient in people with Parkinson's disease.

Dopamine agonists: These are a class of compounds that are similar to dopamine. They bind to dopamine receptors on cells and trigger the same response as dopamine.

Dysarthria: This is an abnormality of speech caused by impairment of the muscles of the mouth and throat that are essential for speaking. It typically manifests as slurred speech.

Dysfunction: Impaired or abnormal function of a specific bodily task. For example, urinary dysfunction refers to any difficulty with urinating.

Dyskinesia: Dyskinesia refers to the excessive movement of muscles in the face or limbs that cannot be controlled voluntarily. In Parkinson's disease, dyskinesias are common complications that develop after seven or eight years of levodopa therapy.

Dysphagia: This refers to difficulty in swallowing or the inability to swallow.

Dysthymia: Dysthymia is a mild, chronic form of depression that is characterized by low energy, decreased self-esteem, sad mood, and tearful episodes.

Dystonia: Dystonia is an involuntary contraction of a single or multiple muscle(s) that causes an abnormal posture. The most common site for dystonia in those with Parkinson's disease is the foot.

Edema: This is swelling caused by the excessive accumulation of fluid in tissues.

Efficacy: Efficacy refers to the extent to which a drug can control the symptoms of a disease.

Encephalopathy: Encephalopathy is a disorder of the brain that can have a variety of causes, resulting in impairment in level of consciousness and/or cognitive abilities.

Enzyme: An enzyme is a protein that accelerates a specific chemical reaction. Enzymes are also essential for the chemical reaction to occur.

Epilepsy: Epilepsy is a neurological disorder in which a person has recurrent, unpredictable seizures.

Erectile dysfunction: Erectile dysfunction is a medical condition in which one is unable to develop or maintain an erection of the penis.

Essential tremor: Essential tremor is the most common type of tremor. It is often confused with the tremor of Parkinson's disease. It occurs mostly in the hands, forearms, and head, when that part of the body is in motion or held in a particular position. The legs and torso are rarely involved.

Euphoria: Euphoria is a state of intense happiness.

Executive function: Executive function is one of the complex, cognitive abilities of humans that covers all of the steps needed for a person to plan and perform complicated tasks.

Festination: This term is used to describe a gait in which someone walks with short, quick, shuffling steps. It is common in Parkinson's disease.

Free radicals: Free radicals are molecules formed as the body goes about its constant task of breaking down food, repairing injuries, maintaining normal metabolism, and so forth. Free radicals are highly reactive and have the potential to cause damage.

Free recall: Free recall is a form of memory in which a specific fact is retrieved without the aid of additional information that may put that fact into context.

Freud, Sigmund: Freud was an Austrian neurologist and psychiatrist who cofounded the psychoanalytic school of psychology. The psychoanalytic school was developed on the hypothesis that the unconscious mind plays a significant role in determining our mood and behaviors.

GABA: GABA is the commonly used abbrevation for the neurotransmitter that is formally known as gamma-aminobutyric acid. It is an inhibitory neurotransmitter that is synthesized and released by cells throughout the brain.

Gait disorder: This is a term that refers to any type of abnormal gait. Parkinson's disease is one of many conditions that result in a gait disorder.

Gene: A gene is composed of DNA molecules and is on a portion of a chromosome. It instructs cells to make a particular protein.

Globus pallidus: The globus pallidus is a portion of the basal ganglia. Experimental evidence suggests that the globus pallidus is overactive in people with Parkinson's disease, sending strong inhibitory messages to the motor cortex of the brain that causes the symptoms of Parkinson's disease. It is the target site for the surgical treatment pallidotomy and one of the sites for deep brain stimulation.

Hallucination: A hallucination is a false perception that occurs without any true sensory stimulus. Visual hallucinations are often described by people with Parkinson's disease and are usually a side effect of Parkinson medications.

Herbicide: This term refers to any compound that is used to kill unwanted plants.

Hesitation: This is the act of pausing. In those with Parkinson's disease, it takes longer than usual to begin a movement. It is the time required to start a movement that is referred to as "hesitation."

Huntington's disease: Huntington's disease is a rare inherited neurological disorder that results in a variety of abnormal movements, psychiatric illness, and dementia.

Hyperkinesia: Hyperkinesia refers to increased, fast motor movement in response to a stimulus. "Hyper" means over, and "kinesis" means movement.

Hypersexuality: This refers to unusual or excessive concern with or indulgence in sexual activity.

Hypertension: Hypertension is a medical condition in which a person's blood pressure is chronically elevated.

Hyperthermia: Hyperthermia is a medical condition in which the body produces or absorbs more heat than it can release, resulting in an excessively elevated body temperature. This is a condition that requires immediate medical attention.

Hypokinesia: Hypokinesia refers to decreased, diminished, or slow motor movement in response to a stimulus. "Hypo" means under, and kinesis means "movement."

Hypomimia: This term is used to indicate decreased facial expression. In Parkinson's disease, the loss of facial expression can be slight, like a "poker face," or completely absent.

Hypophonia: Hypophonia refers to a weak, soft voice. The Lee Silverman Voice Treatment method is sometimes used in Parkinson's disease patients to raise voice volume.

Hypothesis: This is a testable explanation of certain phenomena. For example, in someone who gets frequent headaches and likes to eat chocolate, a hypothesis may be that eating chocolate leads to headaches. This hypothesis can then be tested by having the individual stop eating chocolates and monitor the effect on headaches.

Interpersonal therapy: Interpersonal therapy is a form of psychotherapy that is brief and highly structured. The goal is to define the patient's mood disorder as it relates to his or her relationships with other people. The goal is to change the way in which the patient interacts with other people to improve mood.

Kindred: This is a term that is used to refer to a group of related persons.

Lactulose: Lactulose is a complex sugar. When eaten, it draws water into the bowel, making a person's stool softer and easier to excrete. Lactulose is used to treat constipation.

L-Dopa: People with Parkinson's disease take a drug called levodopa (L-dopa) to replace the dopamine that is missing in their brain. Levodopa is a natural precursor to dopamine and is given in combination with another medication, carbidopa. Levodopa is most effective in reducing tremor, rigidity, and akinesia.

Mania: A psychiatric condition characterized by extremely elevated mood and energy level.

Memory: The ability to store, retain, and subsequently recall information.

Menopause: The physiological cessation of menstrual cycles that is associated with advancing age in women.

Metabolism: This is the basic chemical process that occurs in every cell in every living thing. It is essential for life.

Micrographia: Micrographia refers to small handwriting. In Parkinson's disease, handwriting becomes smaller and more cramped because of the inability to control fine motor movements.

Mitochondria: These are tiny structures inside cells in which the energy needed for metabolism is produced.

Morphology: The study of the outward appearance of a cell, organ, or entire organism.

Motor fluctuations: Motor fluctuations occur after long-term use of L-dopa and refer to a failure of the drug to provide a predictable effect on motor symptoms. The reason for motor fluctuations is poorly understood. They can be predictable ("wearing-off") or unpredictable ("on-off").

MPTP: *N*-methyl-4-phenyl-1,2,3,6-tetrahydropyridine (MPTP) was discovered to cause Parkinson's-like symptoms when illicit drug users created and used it, thinking they had made a version of a narcotic drug. MPTP is now used as a tool in research on the disease.

Multiple system atrophy: This is one of the Parkinson's Plus syndrome diseases. It is a neurodegenerative disease marked by a combination of symptoms affecting movement, blood pressure, and other body functions.

Multitasking: This refers to the ability to perform or supervise the completion of several different jobs or projects at one time.

Mutation: These are changes to the sequence of DNA that result in changes in the protein produced by a given DNA sequence.

Neuron: A neuron is a cell of the nervous system. The brain is made up of many different types of neurons with different functions that are found in different locations of the brain and spinal cord.

Neurotransmission: This term refers to the transfer of signals between neurons.

Neurotransmitter: A neurotransmitter is a chemical that is released from the ending of a neuron. It signals an adjacent nerve or tissue to increase or decrease its activity.

Off period: When someone with Parkinson's disease or a doctor talks about an "off" period, they are referring to a period of time when medication to control the symptoms does not work.

On period: This term describes the time during which someone with Parkinson's disease derives benefit from their medication. It is a period when the disability from Parkinson's symptoms are at a minimum.

Orgasm: Orgasm is part of the sexual response cycle, characterized by intense physical pleasure. It is controlled by the autonomic nervous system.

Orthostatic hypotension: Orthostatic hypotension is a sudden drop in blood pressure that occurs when someone stands up quickly, typically after being in a seated or lying position for an extended period.

Pallidotomy: Pallidotomy is a neurosurgical procedure in which brain cells in the globus pallidus are destroyed. This procedure has been used to treat dyskinesias in those with Parkinson's disease. However, this technique has been largely replaced by the advent of deep brain stimulation.

Parkinson's disease: Parkinson's disease is a progressive disease caused by a deficiency in the chemical production of dopamine in the brain. An individual is diagnosed with Parkinson's disease if they exhibit three of its four cardinal signs. No two patients exhibit the same combination of signs and symptoms, and no two patients progress at the same rate.

Parkinson's Plus syndrome: This refers to a number of similar Parkinson's-like neurodegenerative disorders. The doctor must consider these other conditions when treating a patient. Multiple system atrophy and progressive supranuclear palsy are two examples are of the Parkinson Plus disorders.

Pathology: Pathology is the scientific study of disease processes.

Penetrance: Penetrance is the likelihood that the properties controlled by a specific gene will be expressed.

Pesticide: A pesticide is a substance that is used to prevent, destroy, repel, or lessen the damage of any pest. A pest may be an animal or plant.

PET: PET is an abbreviation for positron emission tomography. This is a non-invasive imaging technique that provides three-dimensional images of the brain and other organs.

Placebo drug: A placebo drug is a medicinal preparation that has no specific pharmacological activity. It is given to a control group in a controlled clinical trial to ensure that the specific effect of the experimental medication can be distinguished from any nonspecific effects. That is, the experimental medication must produce better results than the placebo to be considered effective.

Pluripotent: Some cells are pluripotent, meaning that they have the ability to develop into any number of cell types found throughout the body.

Prevalence: Prevalence refers to the total number of cases of a disease in a specific population at a given time.

Progressive supranuclear palsy: This is one of the Parkinson's Plus syndrome diseases. It is a rare brain disorder that causes serious and permanent problems with control of gait and balance. The most obvious sign of the disease is an inability to voluntarily move the eyes to look up. This occurs because of lesions in the area of the brain that coordinates eye movements.

Protein: A protein is a compound, consisting of amino acids, that is essential in the diet for the growth and repair of tissues of the body.

Psychoanalysis: This is a group of psychological theories that focus on the connections between our unconscious mind and our conscious behaviors. By discovering and understanding these connections, the hope is that one's behaviors can change.

Psychodynamic therapy: This is a form of therapy in which the theories of psychoanalysis are used but for a relatively short period. The goal is to uncover the unconscious concerns and conflicts that are governing specific behaviors. To improve or change those behaviors, the unconscious factors that lead to those behaviors must be identified, understood, and resolved in a way that minimizes the chances that they will cause additional behavioral problems.

Psychosis: Psychosis is a mental disorder characterized by the inability to think clearly, communicate rationally, interact appropriately, and generally understand the surrounding world. Symptoms can be extremely debilitating. Many people with a psychotic disorder get effective relief from antipsychotic medications. Psychotic symptoms include delusions and hallucinations.

Rest tremor: A rest tremor is a tremor that occurs in a body part that is at rest, completely supported against gravity, but does not occur with voluntary movement.

Rigidity: Rigidity is increased stiffness in a muscle when moved by someone else.

Rolfing: Rolfing is a method of soft tissue manipulation in which the goal is to realign the body and make its movement patterns work in a more harmonious manner in relation to gravity.

Schizophrenia: Schizophrenia is a psychiatric illness in which an individual has an impaired perception of reality, resulting in hallucinations and possibly delusions that result in markedly abnormal behavior.

Seizure: A seizure is a temporary, short-term state in which brain cells fire uncontrollably.

Serotonin: This is a neurotransmitter, produced by specific brain cells, that plays an important role in the regulation of mood, level of aggression, and sleep.

Sialorrhea: This word means "drooling," which is quite common in several neurological diseases including Parkinson's. There are several therapies that sometimes control sialorrhea. One therapy is injections of botulinum toxin into one or more salivary glands.

Side effect: A side effect is an undesired outcome of a treatment with a medication or medical procedure.

Sign: A sign is any objective evidence of an illness. Signs are visible to an observer and are independent of a patient's subjective impressions.

SPECT: SPECT is an abbreviation for single photon emission computed tomography. It is a procedure used to study blood flow in various regions of the brain.

Substantia nigra: This is a structure within the basal ganglia of the brain that contains dopamine-producing cells. When these dopamine-producing cells die in sufficient numbers, the result is the development of Parkinson's disease.

Subthalamic nucleus: The subthalamic nucleus is a collection of neurons in the basal ganglia that is involved in regulating movement.

Symptoms: This term refers to the subjective perception an individual has about a change in his or her body. Compare this with a sign, which a doctor can see or measure.

Synapse: A synapse is the specialized region between two nerve cells, in which the chemical communication between them takes place.

Tardive movement disorders: Tardive movement disorders include any abnormality in movement that occurs as a result of exposure to antipsychotic medication. Antipsychotic medications are commonly used to treat psychiatric conditions such as schizophrenia.

Telomere: A telomere is a region of DNA, at the end of each chromosome, that acts to protect the rest of the chromosome from damage.

Thalamotomy: Thalamotomy is a a neurosurgical procedure in which brain cells in the thalamus are destroyed. This procedure has been used to treat tremor in those with Parkinson's disease. However, this technique has been largely replaced with the advent of deep brain stimulation.

Tremor: A tremor is an involuntary movement of a part of the body. A tremor is the result of alternating contractions of opposing muscles.

Urinary incontinence: This refers to the inability to retain urine and the tendency to release small amounts of urine uncontrollably.

Wearing off: "Wearing off" refers to the progressive shortening of the "on" time that follows a dose of L-dopa. Over time, most people, including friends and family, notice that L-dopa therapy works less well, and bradykinesia, tremor, and other symptoms reappear sooner between doses.

Bibliography

Arhey RJ, Porter RW, Walker RW. 2005. Cognitive assessment of a representative community population with Parkinson's disease (PD) using the Cambridge Cognitive Assessment-Revised (CAMCOG-R). *Age and Ageing* 34:268–273.

De Lau LM, Breteler MM. 2006. Epidemiology of Parkinson's disease. *Lancet Neurology* 5:525–535.

Fink JS, Schumacher JM, Ellias SL, Palmer EP, Saint-Hilaire M, Shannon K, Penn R, Starr P, VanHorne C, Kott HS, Dempsey PK, Fischman AJ, Raineri R, Manhart C, Dinsmore J, Isacson O. 2000. Porcine xenografts in Parkinson's disease and Huntington's disease patients: preliminary results. *Cell Transplant* 9:273–278.

Foltynie T, Brayne CEG, Robbins TW, Barker RA. 2004. The cognitive ability of an incident cohort of Parkinson's patients in the UK. The CamPaIGN study. *Brain* 127:550–560.

Goetz CG, Leurgans S, Pappert EJ, Raman R, Stemer AB. 2001. Prospective longitudinal assessment of hallucinations in Parkinson's disease. *Neurology* 57:2078–2082.

Kaeberlein M, Burtner CR, Kennedy BK. 2007. Recent developments in yeast aging. *PLoS Genetics* 3.655–660.

Laun P, Rinnerthaler M, Bogengruber E, Heeren G, Breitenbach M. 2006. Yeast as a model for chronological and reproductive aging—a comparison. *Experimental Gerontology* 41:1208 1212.

Li F, Harmer P, Fisher KJ, Xu J, Fitzgerlad K, Vongjaturapat N. 2007. Tai Chi-based exercise for older adults with Parkinson's disease: a pilot-program evaluation. *Journal of Aging and Physical Activity* 15:139–151.

Paganini-Hill A. 2001. Risk factors for Parkinson's disease: the leisure world cohort study. *Neuroepidemiology* 20:118–124.

Parkinson J. 2002. Essay on the shaking palsy. *Journal of Neuropsychiatry and Clinical Neurosciences* 14:223–236 (original publication, 1817).

Ramig LO, Sapir S, Fox C, Countryman S. 2001. Changes in vocal loudness following intensive voice treatment (LSVT) in individuals with Parkinson's disease: a comparison with untreated patients and normal age-matched controls. *Movement Disorders* 16:79–83.

Redmond Jr DE, Bjugstad KB, Teng YD, Ourednik V, Ourednik J, Wakeman DR, Parsons XH, Gonzalez R, Blanchard BC, Kim SU, Gu Z, Lipton SA, Markakis EA, Roth RH, Elsworth JD, Sladek Jr JR, Sidman RL, Snyder EY. 2007. Behavioral improvement in a primate Parkinson's model is associated with multiple homeostatic effects of human neural stem cells. *Proceedings of the Natonal Academy of Sciences of the United States of America* 104:12175–12180.

Rees PM, Fowler CJ, Mass CP. 2007. Sexual function in men and women with neurological disorders. *Lancet* 369:512–525.

Schuurman AG, van den Akker M, Ensinck KT, Metsemakers JF, Knottnerus JA, Leentjens AF, Buntinx F. 2002. Increased risk of Parkinson's disease after depression. *Neurology* 58:1501–1504.

Shults CW, Oakes D, Kieburtz K, Beal MF, Haas R, Plumb S, Juncos JL, Nutt J, Shoulson I, Carter J, Kompoliti K, Perlmutter JS, Reich S, Stern M, Watts RL, Kurlan R, Molho E, Harrison M, Lew M; Parkinson Study Group. 2002. Effects of coenzyme Q10 in early Parkinson disease: evidence of slowing of the functional decline. *Archives of Neurology* 59:1541–1550.

Tan EK, Tan C, Fook-Chong SM, Lum SY, Chai A, Chung H, Shen H, Zhao Y, Teoh ML, Yih Y, Pavanni R, Chandran VR, Wong MC. 2003. Dose-dependent protective effect of coffee, tea, and smoking in Parkinson's disease: a study in ethnic Chinese. *Journal of the Neurological Sciences* 216:163–167.

Taylor MJ, Freemantle N, Geddes JR, Bhagwagar Z. 2006. Early onset of selective serotonin reuptake inhibitor antidepressant action: systematic review and meta-analysis. *Archives of General Psychiatry* 63:1217–1223.

Von Campenhausen S, Bornschein B, Wick R, Botzel K, Sampaio C, Poewe W, Oertel W, Siebert U, Berger K, Dodel R. 2005. Prevalence and incidence of Parkinson's disease in Europe. *European Neuropsychopharmacology* 15:473–490.

Voukelatos A, Cumming RG, Lord SR, Rossel C. 2007. A randomized, controlled trial of tai-chi for the prevention of falls: the central Sydney tai chi trial. *Journal of the American Geriatrics Society* 55:1185–1191.

Wood-Kaczmar A, Gandhi S, Wood NW. 2006. Understanding the molecular causes of Parkinson's disease. *Trends in Molecular Medicine* 12:521–528.

Index

About the Author

NUTAN SHARMA is on the staff of Massachusetts General Hospital and is an assistant professor at Harvard Medical School. Dr. Sharma was born and raised in western New York state. After completing her clinical training, she joined the staff at Massachusetts General Hospital, where she is currently an assistant neurologist, specializing in the care of individuals with Parkinson's disease and other movement disorders.